Body Language

Body Language

Sisters in Shape,
Black Women's Fitness, and
Feminist Identity Politics

Kimberly J. Lau

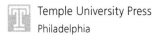
Temple University Press
Philadelphia

TEMPLE UNIVERSITY PRESS
Philadelphia, Pennsylvania 19122
www.temple.edu/tempress

Library of Congress Cataloging-in-Publication Data

Lau, Kimberly J.
  Body language : sisters in shape, black women's fitness, and feminist identity politics /
Kimberly J. Lau.
     p. cm.
  Includes bibliographical references and index.
  ISBN 978-1-4399-0308-7 (cloth : alk. paper) — ISBN 978-1-4399-0309-4
(pbk. : alk. paper) — ISBN 978-1-4399-0310-0 (e-book)
     1. Feminism—United States. 2. Feminist theory—Political aspects. 3. Group
identity—United States. 4. African American women—Social conditions. 5. Self-care,
Health—United States. 6. Women—Socialization—United States. I. Title.
  HQ1181.U5L38 2011
  305.48'896073—dc22

                                                                              2011002813

Printed in the United States of America

121211-P

For Melanie Marchand and the women of Sisters in Shape

Contents

Acknowledgments

One of the ideas that I grapple with in *Body Language* concerns the limitations of language—the moments when language fails us, when our experiences and feelings seem to exceed discourse. This is one of those moments. *Body Language* would not have been possible without the love and labor of many people, and I attempt to thank them here, though I know that words simply cannot convey the extent of my appreciation.

Melanie Marchand and the women of Sisters in Shape have brought this book to life, and I thank them for contributing their voices, their insights, and their stories. I dedicate this book to them, though such a gesture falls far short of my gratitude.

Countless colleagues and friends have also contributed significantly to *Body Language*, some without even realizing it. I have benefited tremendously from critical responses to this project throughout its long life, and I want to start by thanking those whose names I may not even know: the conference, colloquium, and workshop organizers and participants who asked pressing questions and offered useful citations; the graduate students at other universities who offered insights and references after my talks; the anonymous reviewers and readers who so carefully read my work for Temple University Press and for my promotion case, all of whom challenged me in the most productive ways.

In addition, I have been lucky to have colleagues and friends who pushed my thinking and inspired my theorizing and writing in exactly the right ways at exactly the right moments: Dean Mathiowetz, Helene Moglen, Brenda Lyshaug, and Vanita Seth. Their phenomenal intelligence and unbelievable generosity carried me through my most despairing moments and have profoundly enriched *Body Language*. Likewise, Meg Brady, Crystal Parikh, Susie Porter, Cindy Stark, Kathryn Stockton, and Mary Strine all offered important insights and critiques during my time at the University of Utah; at the U.C. Santa Cruz Center for Cultural Studies, Jim Clifford, Chris Connery, Carla Freccero, Susan Gillman, Jodi Greene, Donna Haraway, and David Marriott all asked difficult, challenging, and thus enormously helpful questions.

I also had the pleasure of working with the incomparable Kathy Chetkovich, possibly the smartest, most engaged close reader any writer could ever hope to have. *Body Language* is sharper and clearer because of her commitment to precision in both writing and theorizing, and her friendship made her criticisms seem like a pleasurable conversation over coffee.

At Temple University Press, Janet Francendese has been an exceptional editor—a savvy reader, a thoroughly enjoyable interlocutor, and a gentle guide. Her kindness, humor, and support have been heartening and are deeply appreciated. I also want to thank Charles Ault, Amanda Steele, and Rebecca Logan for helping to bring *Body Language* into being; throughout, their grace and patience have ensured that the process has been both efficient and enjoyable.

This book has been a long time in the making, and during that time I was fortunate to have received institutional support from both the University of Utah and the University of California–Santa Cruz. At the University of Utah, I was awarded a Faculty Fellowship at the Tanner Humanities Center, a Faculty Fellowship from the university, and several grants to support my field research. At the University of California–Santa Cruz, I was awarded several grants from the Committee on Research; this support allowed me to conduct follow-up fieldwork as well as more extensive research with the assistance of Lindsey Collins, a fabulous research assistant who immediately understood the balance of feminist theory and black women's material realities that I was seeking.

I also thank my family and friends for life's comforts, pleasures, and delicacies. And, last, though the words for thanking my partner, John, are truly inadequate, I offer these: refuge, joy, love, life.

Body Language

1 / The Anatomy
of a Movement

On Friday, March 20, 1998, the *Philadelphia Daily News* published an article that would dramatically change the lives of many black women. Written by Marisol Bello and titled "Shape Up, Sisters!" the article offered an extensive portrait of Melanie Marchand, a local fitness professional, and one of her clients, Denise Murphy, who had gone from a size 16 to a size 8 over the course of the previous year and a half. For her article, Bello shadowed Melanie and Denise through one of their typical training sessions, interviewed both of them, and described Melanie's program of weight training, aerobic exercise, and nutrition education in the context of addressing the health problems black women face as a group, including disproportionately high rates of heart disease, diabetes, and obesity. Subtitled "52% of Black Women Overweight," the article caught people's attention. Not only did it offer a snapshot of black women's negative health indicators relative to those of women of other racial and ethnic groups but it also succeeded in capturing Denise's enthusiasm for her lifestyle changes and Melanie's commitment to improving black women's health. At the end of the article, Bello included a short sentence that set everything in motion: "For more information, contact Sisters in Shape."

That day alone, more than one hundred women called Sisters in Shape. More continued to call over the next few days. All told, between two and three hundred women called Sisters in Shape in the week following the article, and the tone of their messages ranged from despair to hope, from anger to motivation. In one of our first interviews, Melanie recalled some of the messages:

> One woman called [raises voice slightly], "I'm three hundred pounds; I'm overweight; I need help; please help me." Another woman [said], "Hi, my name is so-and-so, and I wanna get more information about Sisters in Shape. I'm ready to make a change. I want a new *me*," and she was all excited: "I want a new *me*" [repeated with attitude]. And then you have this other woman who calls and sa[ys], "Hi, my name is so-and-so and me and about five other women here at such-and-such middle school are out of shape and overweight. Please call." It was just really inspiring to hear the hope, the optimism that they had in their voices because they felt like they had found some answer to something that they need help with.

When the calls started, Sisters in Shape was little more than a voice-mail box for three black women who worked as fitness instructors in the city and who performed together as part of the 12th Street Gym aerobics demonstration team. On the basis of their own life experiences and evidence from their classes at a number of gyms in the greater Philadelphia area, Melanie, Kathy Tillery, and Carethia Thomas believed that African American women generally tend not to prioritize exercise and fitness in their lives. Drawing on their collective knowledge, their many years of experience in the exercise and fitness industry, and their status as fitness role models, the three decided to try to increase awareness of the benefits of exercise and nutrition and the importance of living a healthy lifestyle for black women in particular.

The three women named themselves Sisters in Shape and began participating in a number of regional fitness festivals and events, where they would do aerobics demonstrations and then talk to other women, mostly black, about their health and fitness programs and experiences. They came together for annual Philadelphia events such as

Unity Day, Fitness Fest, the City of Hope fitness showcases, smaller health fairs in local churches, and even Power99's radio show *Sistahs*, a program devoted to issues affecting black women's lives. Sisters in Shape was active in the community, but it did not exist as an organization outside these sorts of engagements. Today, almost fifteen years later, Sisters in Shape is one of the most successful health and fitness programs ever developed for black women, with hundreds of longtime members as well as its own gym.

The Politics of Identity Politics

The fact that the *Philadelphia Daily News* article elicited such a response and that Sisters in Shape continues to resonate so deeply with black women reminds us of the ongoing reality and significance of identity to everyday life and politics. What Sisters in Shape's success tells us about the lasting importance of identity, how the group intervenes in feminist theories of identity politics, and why such interventions open up possibilities for alternative models of identity and thus different types of identity politics—these are the primary questions that anchor *Body Language*. The power of Sisters in Shape—first to draw in so many women and then to build a movement in collaboration with them— speaks to the enduring appeal of identity politics even as the group's self-definitions complicate fixed identity categories such as *black women*.

Throughout *Body Language*, I choose to use the term *identity politics* despite the largely hostile and/or dismissive response it often evokes, both as a descriptive term and as a concept, in our supposedly postidentity era. As has become abundantly clear since the early 1990s, identity politics is not without its problems, foremost among them an essentializing impulse and an investment in a fixed sense of the self. Much critiqued by scholars and media pundits on both the right and the left, identity politics has become what Cressida Heyes calls "a philosophical punching bag" ([2002] 2007), and the fact that critics of varying intellectual persuasions generally fail to offer a specific definition of the term they so easily and vociferously attack only facilitates its easy dismissal (see, e.g., Bickford 1997; Jane Martin 1994; Heyes [2002] 2007; and Kruks 2001 for more extensive discussions of this tendency). For many, identity politics has simply become an outdated term and an outmoded concern.[1] Nonetheless, I continue to invoke the term precisely because the women of Sisters in Shape inspire a return to some of the questions that still linger in the shadows of feminist theory and feminist praxis, questions that suggest we may yet find some value in the conceptual and practical underpinnings of identity politics, particularly as they articulate with other theoretical concerns about subjectivity and social change. Along these lines, Susan Bickford's brief overview of some of the most widely circulated meanings of identity politics provides a useful index for understanding the Sisters in Shape women's identity practices: "'Identity politics' can refer to articulating a claim in the name of a particular group; being concerned with cultural specificity, particularly in an ethnic-nationalist sense; acting as though group membership necessitates a certain political stance; focusing to an excessive degree on the psychological; and various combinations of these" (1997: 112). Indeed, each of these meanings is particularly apt for Sisters in Shape and its everyday uses of identity.

Feminist theories of identity formation and identity politics emerge out of many different disciplinary locations even as they intersect at various historical and intellectual junctures. Thus, within "feminist theory," the politics of Sisters in Shape may be seen, from one view, as an affirmation of group experience and a celebration of difference; from another view, the group may just as likely be seen as undermining the its liberatory promise through its investment both in a fixed notion of black womanhood and in a stable and coherent self. The possibility of such polarized interpretations of Sisters in Shape's politics attests to the fraught nature of identity in feminist theories and more broadly.

For women of color, lesbians, and postcolonial feminists, a great deal of liberal, radical, and Western feminist theory depends on universalizing and essentializing impulses. Implicit in such critical analyses of Western feminisms—feminist theories attendant to the social and political concerns of middle-class, white, heterosexual women from the North and West—is a desire to expand the collective experiences that generate both "feminist" theory and "feminist" movements. The now-canonized works of feminists such as Gloria Anzaldúa, Cherríe Moraga, Angela Davis, Audre Lorde, the Combahee River Collective, bell hooks, Chandra Mohanty, and Maria Lugones, as well as the extensive bodies of literature on critical race theory (e.g., Crenshaw 1991; Crenshaw et al. 1995; Williams 1991; Matsuda et al. 1993; Matsuda 1996; Guinier and Torres 2002) and intersectional identity (e.g., Anzaldúa 1987; Davis 1981; Moraga 1983; King 1993; Lorde 1984; Collins 1991, 1998; hooks 1990; V. Smith 1998), all offer valid critiques of hegemonic feminisms and celebrate alternative standpoints as fundamental to any feminist theory based in group identity and collective experience, the dominant method by which liberal and radical Western feminists first articulated their own positions. As a health and fitness project specifically of and for black women and as an organization that makes claims for social recognition and justice for those same women, Sisters in Shape clearly benefits from and participates in black women's identity politics.

At the same time, however, these "difference" feminists—including those who theorize more strategic and fluid models of identity (e.g., Anzaldúa 1990a, 1990b; Spivak 1987; Sandoval 2000)—tacitly assume a unified subject.[2] The transcendental subject of these difference-based feminist theories of identity has, of course, been widely deconstructed by theorists positing postmodern and poststructuralist understandings of the self (most notably Derrida [1974] 1997; Foucault [1972] 1982, [1977] 1995, [1981] 1990; Butler 1990, 1993; and those working in their tradition). Michel Foucault's work has been foundational in establishing the idea that both subject formation and one's sense of one's body occur through discursive practices and power and through the structural effects of language on experience.

Elaborating on Foucault in her well-known work on the "discursive limits of sex," Judith Butler (1993) draws on psychoanalytic theory to suggest that subjectivity and identity are materialized through performative language acts. In theorizing the production of gender through a series of ongoing iterations, Butler's performative theory of gender necessarily calls into question the viability of the standpoint theories elaborated by difference feminists precisely because standpoint theory assumes a stable self whereas performance theorists see the self as being continually (re)produced. Postmodern theories of identity and subjectivity like Butler's call attention to Sisters in Shape's explicit investment in the ostensibly stable category of *black women* as potentially naïve and inattentive to the discursive and disciplinary fields through which their subjectivities are constructed and performed. However, just as postmodern and poststructuralist feminists fault difference feminists for their theoretical commitments to a stable self, difference feminists criticize postmodern theories of identity for the lack of individual agency posited by these radically discursive models of the self.

Even as these largely antithetical theories of identity continue to evolve and their proponents develop finer and finer articulations of their positions, they generally continue to do so in relation to each other. Thus, to try to understand Sisters in Shape's social and political contributions along either of these dominant trajectories is to overlook the complexity the group brings to theoretical discussions of identity and identity politics. *Body Language* instead traces the nuanced and different ways that Sisters in Shape engages in black women's identity politics and, consequently, prompts a reconsideration of feminist identity politics more generally. At the center of the book is an ethnographically based account of the bodily practices and varied discourses through which the Sisters in Shape women construct themselves as a group, articulate and delimit the boundaries of their collective being in relation to prevailing representations of black women, participate in everyday feminist theory making, and rearticulate feminist identity politics. While the Sisters in Shape women's embodied and discursive practices are necessarily constrained by the cultural and material realities of a racist and sexist society—from the controlling images and stereotypes rooted in dominant ideologies to the often inadequate social support, poor housing options, and limited school and work opportunities born of structural inequalities—*Body Language* focuses on the discursive as the site where those realities are interpreted and rearticulated, where the Sisters in Shape women offer their own social and theoretical interventions.

Sisters in Shape: The Emergence of a Movement

In addition to being a health and exercise project for black women, Sisters in Shape is a community, a culture, and a movement—and the co-construction and intersection of these definitions of the group in and against a complex range of popular and theoretical articulations forms the backbone of this book. Sisters in Shape is, in short, a phenomenally successful black women's health and fitness project. Melanie Marchand, the group's founder and driving force, is one of those people who other people want to be.[3] At times she has been a dancer, a competitive bodybuilder, and a model. She is fiercely intelligent and articulate, completely endearing, and down-to-earth, with an easy, hearty laugh and an occasional giggle. She gets a lot done in a day and does it with integrity and style. When I first met her, she was spending her days as one of two marketing directors for Air Products, Inc. (a manufacturer of gases and chemicals for art, medical, food, and industrial applications), a position that combined her backgrounds in chemical engineering and business administration. Late in the evenings and early in the mornings, Melanie did her own weight training, taught aerobics and other fitness classes, and trained clients. Squeezed into and between work, fitness, and fitness work (teaching and training others) were her other engagements, most of them reflective of her commitments to encouraging and mentoring other African Americans in the various communities of which she is a part—representing her company at professional meetings like that of the National Society of Black Engineers, for instance, or choreographing pieces for the annual show at the W.E.B. Du Bois College House at the University of Pennsylvania while she was working on her master's in business administration at Penn's Wharton School.

In the late 1980s, when Melanie began teaching aerobics in Philadelphia—both at the University of Pennsylvania and at gyms throughout the city—she noticed that the small number of black women in her classes was highly disproportionate to the city's, and even the university's, demographics. Talking with other black fitness instructors in the city, she learned that black women were largely absent from their classes as well, a finding supported by research on physical activity and exercise among women of color. The Centers for Disease Control, for instance, has found that fewer than 30 percent of women of color in the United States get enough physical activity to derive health benefits (cited in Henderson and Ainsworth 2001; see also Wells 1996 and Young et al. 1998). Thus, although black women have had a longtime presence in women's athletics (see, e.g., Cahn 1994; Vertinsky and Captain 1998; Captain 1991; Gissendanner 1994; Y. Smith 1992; Lansbury 2001; and Dumas 2004) and are among the most iconic female athletes, a relatively small percentage of black women participate in noncompetitive exercise and fitness.

The local picture began to change with the *Philadelphia Daily News* article. The organizational story of how Sisters in Shape grew from an

initial group of three committed fitness enthusiasts into its current con-
figuration as one of the most successful health and fitness programs
ever developed for black women is a testament to Melanie's vision as
well as to many other women's overwhelming desire for information
and change where health and their bodies are concerned. When the
calls started streaming in to the Sisters in Shape voicemail box, Melanie
wanted to respond to each and every woman even though she realized
the virtual impossibility of such a task. Instead, she decided the best
strategy would be to hold a free Sisters in Shape health and fitness symposium. The resulting Sunday afternoon event was designed to address
black women's health from an integrated perspective: two medical doctors discussed black women's poor health statistics and the ways that
exercise and balanced nutrition might help redress some of those health
conditions, an herbalist talked about alternative treatments and herbal
supplements, an exercise scientist commented on the overall benefits of
exercise and fitness, a spiritual consultant offered insight into the relationship between bodily well-being and spiritual health, and a motivational speaker helped structure the whole event and encouraged women
to commit to making major lifestyle changes.

A Different Kind of "Strong Black Woman"

At the symposium, Melanie called attention to—and dismissed—some
of the culturally specific excuses black women use to rationalize their
lack of exercise. "Do not tell me that you spent too much money having your hair straightened and sweat will ruin it," she scolded. "Do not
tell me you can't afford to join a gym or to work with a personal trainer
when you're spending hundreds of dollars a week having your hair and
nails done," she added. (Sisters in Shape has always operated on a sliding scale and even secured special Sisters in Shape rates from its original sponsor, 12th Street Gym.) "Do not tell me that your man likes you
big," she continued. "Do not tell me that greens have to be cooked with
a fat ham hock to taste good." The women in the audience laughed
knowingly, nodded enthusiastically, and seemed to take a certain pleasure in being called out. More than an admonishment, Melanie's good-
natured dismissal of these excuses helped create the sense that Sisters
in Shape was, indeed, a health and fitness project devoted specifically

to black women and their needs, and the almost two hundred women present got the message.

Once the laughter subsided, Melanie tackled one of the biggest obstacles to black women's widespread participation in exercise programs: taking (or making) the time to prioritize themselves. While competing demands on one's time and attention affect women of all races and ethnicities, the cultural power of the myth of the strong black woman compounds this problem for black women. Unlike dominant stereotypical representations of black women as mammies, Sapphires, and Jezebels,[4] the image of the strong black woman has been positively accepted within black communities and fetishized by the larger society. And yet, as black feminist critics have pointed out, the idea of the strong black woman is a complex one that recognizes historical legacies of survival and resistance while also creating impossible standards for everyday life (see, e.g., Wallace [1978] 1990; Gillespie [1978] 1984; Harris 1995, 2001; Harris-Lacewell 2001; Beauboeuf-Lafontant 2005, 2007, 2009; Romero 2000; C. Thompson 2000; Dorsey 2002; Thomas, Witherspoon, and Speight 2004; Woods-Giscombé 2010). Further, the image is often naturalized and internalized among black women such that they measure themselves against an ideal of superhuman capabilities—the ability to care for everyone, to hold everything together, to solve everyone's problems. Obviously, the strong black woman does not have much time for herself; nor—as the myth would have it—does she need much time. As a result, many black women express concerns over being perceived as selfish or "unduly focused on the self" if they limit their roles as extensive physical and emotional caretakers and problem solvers (Beauboeuf-Lafontant 2007: 41).

With an intimate understanding of such concerns, Melanie emphasized the fact that taking care of other people requires taking care of oneself first. Over time, this has become one of Sisters in Shape's central tenets, and it speaks to the physical and emotional consequences of trying to live the myth of the strong black woman. As sociologist Tamara Beauboeuf-Lafontant has demonstrated, the myth of the strong black woman has serious implications for black women's physical and emotional health (2005, 2007, 2009). Through her interviews, Beauboeuf-Lafontant found that many women sought to hide or "internalize" their "strength-discrepant realities and feelings," and this "internalization took form in behaviors, including overindulging in eating, shopping, and drinking, as well as in physical and mental distress, namely, hypertension, heart disease, stomach ills, respiratory difficulties, and depressive episodes, often referred to as nervous breakdowns" (2007: 36). Recognizing the power of such expectations and controlling images, Melanie explicitly gave the women present permission to care for themselves as a fundamental way of caring for others. In so doing, she also demonstrated that Sisters in Shape understands and embraces the nuanced and particular complexities of black women's relationships to others as well as to the material realities that constrain their exercise practices and their attention to themselves.

Even more, Sisters in Shape transforms the strong black woman from a controlling discourse to a physical incarnation, thus providing an alternative way for women to hold on to the positive, resistant aspects of the image. That is, Melanie's heavily muscled body continues to represent the value of strength but in a way that contests the unreasonable expectations implicit in the myth of the black superwoman while also consolidating Sisters in Shape's prioritization of the self. Within this context, the black woman's strong body insists on being seen, and this demand for recognition—of not only the body but also the self—is a critical rearticulation of a controlling image and dangerous myth. As gender and sports scholar Leslie Heywood has argued in her work on female bodybuilders, the "sovereignty inherent in bodybuilding" (1998: 170) and the ways it "recuperates to-be-looked-at-ness" (159) disturb dominant gender ideologies and unsettle long-standing assumptions about women's subjectivity: "Women's bodybuilding is an unequivocal self-expression, an indication of women's right to *be*, not for children, partners, fellow activists, not for anyone else" (171). While Sisters in Shape is not exactly a women's bodybuilding organization, the women's muscled bodies similarly represent a mode of cultural activism and open up new ways of imagining the strong black woman.

Building a Movement, Creating a Community

While it is obvious that Melanie is a symbol of strength, a committed fitness role model, and a charismatic leader with a contagious and inspirational energy, it is equally clear that Sisters in Shape is unique as a health and fitness project for black women because of its broad grass-roots appeal and collective sense of ownership. In the first few months following the symposium, Sisters in Shape began offering monthly educational workshops—covering such topics as the benefits of weight training, how to work aerobic exercise into a daily schedule, and the use of nutrition to boost metabolism—as well as group exercise events such as weekly power walks along Martin Luther King Jr. Drive (the West River Drive) and Cardio-Funk step aerobics classes. Meeting in these contexts helped solidify a feeling of community among the first women to join Sisters in Shape, and it is actually many of these women who built an organization out of a service. Typical of this early transformation, the first Sisters in Shape aerobics demonstration after the symposium involved not just Melanie and Kathy (Carethia had already left the group to devote more time to her own fitness career) but also half a dozen other Sisters in Shape members at varying stages of meeting their fitness goals. In the true spirit of a grassroots organization, Sisters in Shape continued to grow according to the interests and skills of its earliest members: one added a monthly newsletter, another helped with a web page, and a third began circulating recipes for nutritionally balanced traditional foods.

As many different women participated in the slow transformation of Sisters in Shape into a community and not just a fitness program, Melanie also gave herself over to the incredible demand. Within days of the symposium, she left her lucrative corporate job (opting, instead, to work as a part-time contractor for the same company) so she could devote herself to developing Sisters in Shape (itself a full-time job, especially after Kathy's departure a few months later). Within a year, Melanie had quit even her contract work. Sisters in Shape became her only job and the focus of all her time, energy, and marketing savvy.

Now, more than ten years later, in addition to its slate of ongoing classes, Sisters in Shape produces an annual Health and Fitness Explosion, a daylong program of exercise and education that attracts more than five hundred women. Smaller subsets of the group—the "core members"—also appear as fairly regular guest fitness experts on a local television morning show, where they demonstrate various aerobic exercises, weight-lifting techniques, and stretches. Melanie has also collaborated with the Einstein Heart Institute to offer free satellite versions of

Sisters in Shape in Germantown, an outlying neighborhood of Philadelphia. This twelve-week program was the most popular health education program ever sponsored by the Einstein Medical Centers,[5] and many of the participants later joined Sisters in Shape. Most important, however, is Melanie's new Sisters in Shape gym, a physical space that continues to cultivate the sense of community at the center of the organization.

Coming Together as a Real Community

Sisters in Shape engages women collectively as well as individually, and thus it is both a real community and an imagined one. The real community is a face-to-face one, a group of women who come together at different times for different reasons: to celebrate and affirm, to empower and discuss, and to practice and share the lifestyle choices they have made through the Sisters in Shape philosophy. They come together to exercise, to eat, and to talk; they meet for Sisters in Shape events and for movies, sports, shopping, and even vacations. They are a community of women and a community of friends, and this—together with the strength of the Sisters in Shape imagined community—is what distinguishes them from other weight-loss programs and from other twelve-step groups.

Sisters in Shape really began in earnest with the 1998 *Philadelphia Daily News* article and the subsequent health and fitness symposium, and to this day the annual Sisters in Shape Health and Fitness Explosion continues to provide the same community outreach and energy. The Health and Fitness Explosion also offers the best overarching structure for describing what Sisters in Shape does as an organization. This daylong event attracts approximately five hundred to six hundred women, almost all of whom are black. The event, with fees of $50 to $70 (which includes a new pair of Nike aerobics shoes for the first hundred women who register), consists of six breakout sessions, half devoted to different types of exercise (both aerobic and anaerobic) and half devoted to health, nutrition, and "empowerment" education (including such topics as self-esteem, spirituality, and stress reduction). In addition, there are usually two plenary sessions, one that addresses different aspects of black women's disproportionately poor health statistics in this country and one that varies according to the speaker's area of expertise. In the past, plenary speakers have included doctors, entertainers, writers, and motivational speakers. At noon, all participants come together for a luncheon at which the Sisters in Shape core members share their stories, offer aerobics demonstrations, and honor "the most inspirational" Sisters in Shape member of the year. Also on hand are wellness practitioners (including Western biomedical doctors, psychotherapists, massage therapists, chiropractors, and alternative healers) and a handful of vendors selling African and African-inspired clothing; self-help and other empowerment books and publications; and handmade soaps, lotions, and oils. The event is festive, and the participants are generally overwhelmingly energetic despite having spent hours in multiple exercise classes that may have included African dance, belly dancing, Brazilian samba, kickboxing, funk- or hip-hop-inspired aerobics, yoga, and Pilates.

All of this runs smoothly thanks to the Sisters in Shape core members, who set up and decorate the group's designated space at the Philadelphia Convention Center, help register participants in the morning, move women along to the proper breakout rooms, coordinate the luncheon, offer information, sell T-shirts and memberships, and share their own personal histories with women who may be curious about making similar lifestyle changes. The Sisters in Shape core members are living models for the program. Many have been members since the beginning. Some have lost more than a hundred pounds of fat and replaced some of that weight with muscle; some have dropped in dress size from 18 or 20 or 24 to 8 or 10 or 12. They have slowly lost inches upon inches and kept them off for five, six, seven, and even ten years. Many have lowered their blood pressure and cholesterol levels dramatically; others have had major surgeries such as double hip replacement and come back to exercise with the group within the year. Their stories are a fundamental part of the Sisters in Shape organizational narrative, and the annual Health and Fitness Explosion is just one of many opportunities to (re)construct and narrate the group's history.

While the Health and Fitness Explosion is the most visible, public way in which Sisters in Shape comes together as a physical community, the Sisters in Shape women create and sustain their community through face-to-face interactions in many other contexts as well. Early on, when Sisters in Shape was just forming, members met below the Philadelphia Museum of Art before heading off to walk Martin Luther

King Jr. Drive together. In addition to providing obvious health benefits, these walks helped cement many of the social relationships and friendships that characterize Sisters in Shape today, drawing women together for exercise, support, and companionship. At the time, Sisters in Shape was working in collaboration with 12th Street Gym, where Melanie taught a number of aerobics classes, and her classes, in particular, offered another opportunity for Sisters in Shape members to build community.

Many of Melanie's Cardio-Funk step aerobics classes were well known to everyone who used the gym because of the involvement of the Sisters in Shape women who took them, congregating on one side of the room and encouraging each other as well as everyone else in the class with their call-and-response-style interactions with Melanie. In this windowless room, their energy seemed to reverberate off the walls, increasing the noise level to the point where the class was likely heard in the basketball court one floor down; their energy was contagious, and even in the midst of the hardest set of lunges, I could not repress a smile as the Sisters in Shape women counted off the lunges with Melanie. I have never been in an aerobics class anywhere—San Francisco, Berkeley, Oakland, Southern California, Salt Lake City, or Philadelphia (including other classes taught by Melanie)—where participants have been so enthusiastically engaged with the instructor, the class, and the other members.

Today, Sisters in Shape has its own gym, and many of those early Cardio-Funk class regulars work there part-time, for the social and community benefits as well as for the extra income. The new Sisters in Shape gym extends and expands the community-based spirit of the early aerobics classes. Not only do Sisters in Shape members work at the new gym; they also have the opportunity to take many more classes together. In this way, the physical space of their own gym fosters a greater sense of real, lived community as there are many more options for group exercise. At 12th Street Gym, Melanie's classes slowly became Sisters in Shape classes, but there were always Sisters in Shape members whose schedules prevented them from attending those specific group classes; instead, they chose individual ways of getting their cardiovascular workouts (interestingly, they rarely took other instructors' aerobics classes if they could not make the Sisters in Shape classes with Melanie). Now, however, Sisters in Shape members have tremendous flexibility in terms of taking classes with other Sisters in Shape members. Without question, the new gym functions as a community center for the women of Sisters in Shape, a physical site where they can meet to exercise, to talk, or simply to hang out with each other—a powerful new social institution where they can see themselves reflected back in the bodies and the language of the others around them.[6]

Even before Sisters in Shape opened its own gym, Melanie helped create an environment and a schedule that distinguished Sisters in Shape from the general atmosphere of 12th Street Gym. For instance, on Saturday mornings, Sisters in Shape members had their own special ninety-minute exercise class, the genre of which changed from week to week. Guest instructors taught activities as varied as Brazilian samba, kickboxing, belly dancing, yoga, African dance, and Pilates, and the Sisters in Shape women shimmied and kicked and rolled their bellies with good humor and incredible energy. For many, these classes set the mood for the rest of the day, which became a scaled-down version of the annual Health and Fitness Explosions. After the special Sisters in Shape class, many women either took a break to get something to eat or lifted weights or just hung out with friends until it was time for Melanie's ninety-minute Cardio-Funk step aerobics class. From there, they went to Melanie's sixty-minute Final Cut class, a group weight-lifting class, and then they sometimes grabbed another quick bite before reconvening for an afternoon rap session with other Sisters in Shape members. These sessions addressed topics such as blood health and cholesterol concerns, cooking for family gatherings, keeping fit while injured, and eating while on vacation. Many of the Sisters in Shape members spent all of Saturday in the gym, going from one class to another with only short breaks to eat and to chat with friends and fellow members. Of course, not all members participated in all classes, and attendance varied from week to week, but usually between fifteen and twenty-five Sisters in Shape members were present throughout the day. Thus, by the end of any given Saturday, the women of Sisters in Shape had successfully reaffirmed and reestablished their community in the midst of a downtown Philadelphia gym.

During the week, Sisters in Shape members tended toward more individual workout schedules and gym routines, though Melanie's midweek classes at 12th Street Gym were always considered Sisters in Shape events by the members. Now that Sisters in Shape has its own gym, every day is much more like Saturday at 12th Street Gym, though a bit toned down. Most women do not have the time (or the strength and stamina) to take every single class, attend every rap session, and hang out at the gym with other Sisters in Shape women, but because this is their space, the overall tenor captures the spirit and energy of those early Saturdays at 12th Street Gym.

In addition to taking classes, talking through the Sisters in Shape philosophy, and working and playing together, the Sisters in Shape women also offer classes and fitness demonstrations for audiences at local events, at health fairs, and even on morning television shows. They have been featured in national magazines such as *Heart and Soul* and *Ladies' Home Journal*. For these demonstrations and publicity events, they not only practice specific aerobic routines and exercises but also coordinate costumes and help each other with hair and makeup in ways that foster an even deeper sense of group identity.

This structure—the group classes, the rap sessions, the socializing, the team demonstrations, and now the Sisters in Shape gym—distinguishes Sisters in Shape from other group weight-loss programs such as Jenny Craig and Weight Watchers as well as from other support groups such as Alcoholics Anonymous. While these other programs and groups often have their own spaces, meet regularly, and share beliefs and practices, they tend to be organized predominantly for daily support and for education (at least insofar as this furthers the support paradigm) but rarely for socializing beyond the immediate group meeting (more traditional twelve-step programs such as Alcoholics Anonymous are something of an exception because of the mentor model at their core, but again, most of those relationships are devoted to supporting recovery from addiction). Sisters in Shape goes far beyond a support paradigm, though the group structure certainly makes lifestyle changes easier to incorporate in a lasting way. In keeping with the group's tendency to reorient dominant discourses, Sisters in Shape prioritizes overall health and social empowerment in ways that tend to remove "weight loss" from the group's explicit goals; as a result, institutional "support" as an explicit discursive focus tends to recede, becoming a secondary concern.

An Imagined Community Worth Not Dying For

Like the nation as imagined community, Sisters in Shape's imagined community is sustained by shared information and beliefs, common cultural practices and rituals, and unifying foundational and ideological narratives. As Benedict Anderson made clear in first describing the rise of nation-states as imagined communities (1983), the ability to understand oneself as part of a larger social collectivity with similar beliefs is powerful enough to die for, and while Sisters in Shape's imagined community does not inspire the patriotic loyalty of many nation-states, it does fulfill some of our deepest desires for belonging in a fractured, postmodern world. Even more, for the Sisters in Shape women, real community and imagined community closely overlap in a way that extends the power and appeal of each.

Together with the ways in which Sisters in Shape functions as a "real" community, the basic Sisters in Shape principles provide a framework within which women participate in various individual ways and on many different levels. Such principles relate to eating and nutrition, exercise and wellness, and spirituality and friendship. Perhaps most important, the consistency and simplicity of the Sisters in Shape principles—not to mention the degree to which most women seem to internalize them—and the strength of Sisters in Shape's collective identity also create a powerful imagined community for the group's members.

When a woman first joins Sisters in Shape, she usually meets with Melanie for a new-client orientation. At this session, Melanie discusses the woman's health and fitness goals with her, introduces her to the Sisters in Shape nutritional guidelines, establishes an exercise routine, and takes body measurements (both body fat percentages and bicep, waist, and thigh circumferences). The woman leaves with an eating plan—some combination of complex carbohydrates, ample amounts of low-fat protein, plenty of fresh vegetables (cooked without salt or butter), fruit and natural fruit juices (though not after 3:00 p.m.), and lots of water. While eating plans are tailored to each woman's specific needs and issues, they are all based on the same nutritional principles. Therefore, all Sisters in Shape members commit to the same foundations of nutrition, understand the reasoning behind the group's nutritional practices, and ultimately share a commitment to this lifestyle with the other members in the group, thereby contributing significantly to Sisters in Shape as an imagined community.

In general, Sisters in Shape encourages women to eat. Fear of food is a problem for a number of the women who participate in Sisters in Shape—the residue of previous unsuccessful diets, eating disorders, and disordered eating that affect so many women of all ethnicities in the United States[7]—and these women often associate eating with negative body feelings and being overweight. Thus, nutritional counseling and education are crucial to overall health and can help women with poor eating habits, including those who simply fear food. The Sisters in Shape nutritional philosophy emphasizes the relationship between food and energy and demands that women eat regularly, often, and in sufficient quantity to provide their bodies with "fuel" for vigorous exercise.

A new Sisters in Shape member also leaves her orientation with a personally tailored exercise regimen that takes into consideration her goals; her time to exercise in relation to her other commitments; her cardiovascular, muscular, and overall body health; and her sense of what she can afford and where she may fit on Sisters in Shape's sliding scale (e.g., in addition to how much she can pay for any given service, she may also consider whether she wants a monthly or annual gym membership, weekly personal weight training, monthly meetings with Melanie or another Sisters in Shape trainer to work out the next month's plan, etc.). Some women have the time and resources for plans that include five days of cardiovascular workouts and three days of weight training with a personal trainer; others do between three and five days of cardio coupled with one day of personal training and another day of weight lifting on their own. The combinations are virtually endless. Some women try to take advantage of all the group exercise classes, while others prefer to run on the treadmill or ride the stationary bike; still others try to strike a balance between individual and group exercise. The same goes for weight training—some women train regularly, up to three times a week (with Melanie or another Sisters in Shape personal trainer); some who have the financial resources choose to do so in their own homes; some lift just as often but less frequently with a trainer; and some choose to strength-train only in the group exercise classes. While there are no strict Sisters in Shape requirements to weight-train, strength training is a major component in the group's philosophy, mainly because of the metabolic advantages of greater muscle mass and the potential increases in bone density from weight lifting.

Each Sisters in Shape woman also keeps her own exercise and eating log in which she records her workouts and her meals as well as any other notes she wishes to make. On the surface, this personal account appears to be a simple means of record keeping, but the exercise and eating log goes well beyond that, as it also functions as a discursive space in which Melanie and the Sisters in Shape member interact. If the woman has a regular personal trainer—most likely Melanie—they read through the book together whenever they meet, discussing the entries, and the trainer records the weight-lifting session in the book. The trainer may also write notes to the woman—what to eat more of, what to consider in terms of aerobic exercise, when to rest, and so on. In essence, the log is both part of the real face-to-face community and part of the structure of the Sisters in Shape imagined community. Between sessions with Melanie—whether weight-lifting sessions or monthly nutritional consultations—women can engage in real and imaginary dialogue with her (or with their Sisters in Shape trainer) by writing in their logs. At the same time, because virtually all of the Sisters in Shape women keep logs, they can also imagine themselves in common practice with other group members. Even at the most basic levels, Sisters in Shape understands discourse as crucial to body wellness and overall health.

Commonalities such as these—shared understandings of the Sisters in Shape nutritional guidelines, the commitment to keep exercise and eating logs, and similar goals for living a healthy life—foster a true sense of group identity and bolster the Sisters in Shape imagined community. In addition, Sisters in Shape has a monthly newsletter and a website with a guest book that serves, to some degree, as an interactive forum, and both further contribute to the maintenance of Sisters in Shape as simultaneously an imagined and a real community (as Anderson [1983] has argued with respect to the rise of nation-states, print culture and print capitalism were fundamental to the creation of the nation as an imagined community). The Sisters in Shape newsletter features a column by Melanie, details Sisters in Shape members' stories, offers recipes and health and exercise tips, introduces new classes, and provides information about upcoming Sisters in Shape events. In addition to its informational and inspirational aspects, the newsletter provides a connection to Sisters in Shape for women who may not be able to join the Sisters in Shape gym, may not have time to attend many of the group exercise classes, or do not have the option of working with a personal trainer. For these women—as well as for the core members—the Sisters in Shape newsletter allows them to perceive themselves as part of a larger community of black women striving to live healthy lives in a culture that often renders them silent and invisible.

For the women of Sisters in Shape, both the real and the imagined are fundamental to their sense of themselves as a distinct and unique community. Sisters in Shape as a real community provides the social underpinnings for the major lifestyle changes these women seek to make, while Sisters in Shape as an imagined community offers a constant, everyday sense of belonging, a group identity predicated on their own empowerment, strength, and choices for healthy living. Not surprisingly, the Sisters in Shape imagined community also eases the challenges of new eating practices and new exercise regimens, especially for women whose families, friends, coworkers, or other communities simply do not understand their choices. Such support in the form of imagined community is common among weight-loss and recovery programs, but in many cases support slides quickly into discipline, especially for groups whose sole purpose is "weight loss" or "recovery." While support undoubtedly takes on some of these disciplinary and regulatory aspects for the Sisters in Shape women, the spirit of the real community diminishes the likelihood of support as primarily disciplinary. Rather, the friendship, empathy, and sheer enjoyment of each other's company that emerges in the real community facilitates an imagined community worth *not* dying for, a community based on health, fitness, and spirituality.

These real and imagined communities are also fundamental to Sisters in Shape as a social movement—the process through which a group of people first comes to understand its experiences and interests as collective as well as culturally, socially, and structurally determined and constrained and then begins to develop a political analysis that it seeks to share with others whom it sees as embedded in similar circumstances. As I use the term, *social movement* need not index an especially widespread or contentious collective effort but refers more specifically to a set of shared practices and beliefs premised on social solidarity, group incorporation, and ongoing progress toward an alternative future. In this regard, my definition differs from the well-established sociological and political science understandings of social movements that emphasize formal and/or contentious engagements with public politics (e.g., Tilly 1978, 2004; Tarrow 1994). At the same time, my definition follows in the tradition of new social movement theories that implicitly prioritize social change based on identity and culture over political economy, although such theories obviously see the two as mutually constitutive (e.g., Larana, Johnston, and Gusfield 1994; Offe 1985; Freeman and Johnson 1999).

Within this context, I use the term *activism* to refer to the actions and interventions that groups (and individuals within groups) undertake to articulate and share their political analysis to bring about the alternative future they desire. In suggesting that the Sisters in Shape women's discourses and bodily practices are the activisms that enable their social movement, *Body Language* takes up questions posed by gender and sport scholars about the degree to which politicized body projects might subvert and/or resist social, cultural, and historical oppressions (see, e.g., Heywood 1998; Heywood and Dworkin 2003; Dworkin and Messner 1999; and Dworkin and Wachs 2009). In their work on the production of normative gender through sport, Shari L. Dworkin and Michael A. Messner capture the complexity at the center of such questions by highlighting both the potentially liberating aspects of women's participation in sport and the ways that media representations limit such potential through a commodified feminism, a corporate sense of empowerment, and hegemonic standards of femininity (1999). In *Bodymakers: A Cultural Anatomy of Women's Bodybuilding*, Heywood similarly zeroes in on the issues at stake when she asks, "Will images of strong women help women in general be strong? Does physical strength have any relation—other than imagined—to our power and strength in the social world?" (1998: 191). For the Sisters in Shape women, I believe that the answers to these questions can only be yes. That is, the group's everyday bodily praxis is an ongoing activism that disrupts the material reality of black women's disproportionately negative health status, while their discursive framing of that activism reimagines and rearticulates black women's subjectivity and presence in a racist and sexist culture, altering their "power and strength in the social world."

The Women of Sisters in Shape

Despite a common theoretical orientation toward activism and shared goals for black women's health, the individual women of Sisters in Shape have widely divergent backgrounds and experiences. Because the particulars of their lives contribute to their social and material realities and their various standpoints, I offer a sketch of the group's diversity in an effort to help contextualize the ways in which the Sisters in Shape women originate their own theoretical interpretations and positions.

Though the Sisters in Shape membership totals in the hundreds, I know only forty to forty-five of the most regular members, having interviewed about twenty-five of the women at least once during my fieldwork. Over the course of five years I worked closely with about a dozen women, Sisters in Shape "core" members, a designation conferred by Melanie to identify women who have taken on organizational responsibilities and leadership roles, who act as spokeswomen and performers for the group, and who provide Sisters in Shape with a consistent presence and structure. The following demographic sketch comes from direct interview questions as well as from information gleaned from shared conversations with these women (both on tape and off), information passed along by other women, and information provided by Melanie. It is not a statistical representation of all the Sisters in Shape members; nor is it a statistical representation of Sisters in Shape core members. Rather, it is an attempt to convey some sense of who these women are (in terms of their ages, work, levels of education, class backgrounds, sexuality, and family and relationship status) and to give further depth to their discourse.

The Sisters in Shape women range in age from early 20s to early 60s, though most are somewhere in their late 30s to late 40s. The women represented throughout *Body Language* are quite evenly divided by age, with Allison, Katrina, and LaTanya in their 20s; Nicole, Justine, and Toni in their 30s; Charlie, Bev, Joi, Cassandra, and Miriam in their 40s; and Sonja in her 50s.[8] Of these twelve women, almost half have children (Allison, Justine, Charlie, Cassandra, and Sonja), and of those with children, one is a single, heterosexual working mother (Justine); the others with children have male partners or grown children who have already moved away from home. Most of these women are in heterosexual relationships or have expressed a desire to be in a heterosexual relationship, and only one self-identified as a lesbian, which seems largely consistent with Sisters in Shape members generally. As such, most of these Sisters in Shape women live in fairly traditional nuclear-family settings or in heterosexual domestic partnerships, with few having other domestic arrangements, such as living with and serving as the primary caregiver for elderly parents (Sonja) or living with a sibling's nuclear family (Miriam).

While family background is often a greater indicator of class status and class background than work and income, all three (class, family background, and work) seem fairly interrelated among this group of twelve women, who are solidly middle class and, in one or two cases, might be considered upper middle class. These women's job titles include executive assistant, office manager for a small business, dental hygienist, management consultant, school counselor, and Philadelphia jails employee, positions that mostly depend on a middle-class trajectory of high school and college educations. Other Sisters in Shape members have careers as television news reporters and news anchors, lawyers, nationally recognized musicians, public health educators, accountants, social workers, software engineers, journalists, music promoters, foundation directors, public relations specialists, business owners, beauticians, sales clerks, and office workers. A rare few do the unpaid domestic labor of childrearing and housework (including several who are partnered with NBA stars who play for the Philadelphia 76ers).

One of the cornerstones of the Sisters in Shape program is its financial accessibility, as the group offers a sliding scale for fees and services including membership dues and personal training sessions. Nonetheless, Sisters in Shape still seems to attract mainly middle-class and upper-middle-class women, along with a small number of working-class women, all of whom have the luxury of time in addition to the benefit of disposable income.[9] Thus, while this range of careers and jobs implies a fairly high level of education among the Sisters in Shape members (I estimate that two-thirds to three-quarters of the women are college educated, with another 10 to 15 percent holding advanced degrees), this trend makes sense within the context of Sisters in Shape, a program that attracts women who have not only the time and resources to devote to personal health and wellness but also the educational and class backgrounds that privilege such prioritizations.

Keeping Up with Sisters in Shape: A Note on Fieldwork

Keeping pace with Sisters in Shape is nearly impossible, as I learned during my years doing fieldwork with them. While I was living in Philadelphia, my fieldwork was consistent with more conventional understandings of what constitutes such research: I participated in the daily life of an emerging grassroots health and fitness project for black women, which I knew about through my personal relationship with Melanie.[10] Six months into the project, however, I moved to Salt Lake City, where I began a job at the University of Utah. From that time forward, fieldwork consisted of extended weekend trips to Philadelphia, about once every six to eight weeks, with more frequent and/or longer visits in the summers.

Those weekend fieldwork visits quickly began to fit a set structure—dinner with Melanie on one of the first nights I was in town, followed by a full day of participant observation and interviewing on Saturday, and then dinner with Melanie on Saturday night or breakfast together on Sunday morning. Saturday's routine began with the 8:30 a.m. Sisters in Shape class (which might be Brazilian samba, kickboxing, or yoga), followed by interviews from 10:00 to 11:45 a.m., Cardio-Funk step aerobics from 11:45 to 1:15, the Final Cut weight-lifting class from 1:15 to 2:15, lunch with Melanie and other Sisters in Shape members, interviews from 3:30 to about 6:00 p.m., and then, often, dinner with Melanie (or a return to my hotel room to shower and crash for the night). Mixed into this schedule—Thursday, Friday, and sometimes Sunday—were interviews with Sisters in Shape members who did not come to any of Saturday's classes.

My fieldwork involved both participant observation and interviewing, even though participation in Sisters in Shape activities rarely felt like "work," with the possible exception being a few early morning Brazilian samba classes. A bit self-conscious about my lack of rhythm and my inability to shake my butt while walking and shimmying my shoulders, I admit that I found the samba classes particularly difficult, though not without their hilarity. Similarly, despite my elevated heart rate and intense muscle burn brought on by the Cardio-Funk step aerobics class and the Final Cut weight-lifting class, both activities felt more like social events than work—times to free the body even as we try to discipline it—with lots of whooping and hollering and laughing.

I also participated in a number of non-exercise-based Sisters in Shape events, including some of the semiregular seminars devoted to specific topics such as using herbs for overall health or boosting metabolism through nutrition. One of the largest Sisters in Shape social events was an intimate afternoon with jazz artist Wynton Marsalis, Melanie's childhood sweetheart and longtime friend, who gave a motivational speech about setting and achieving goals. Participating in this event was not only thoroughly enjoyable and entertaining—in addition to talking, Marsalis also played a few tunes on his trumpet—but also important because it helped me establish an organizational identity as someone central to Sisters in Shape. The core Sisters in Shape members ensured that the event ran smoothly, and my participation (mostly helping Melanie in whatever capacity she needed) was both central and visible. Moreover, many of the Sisters in Shape women also understood that my flying to Philadelphia from Salt Lake City specifically for this event showed a serious commitment to Sisters in Shape generally. Similarly, my regular presence at the annual Sisters in Shape Health and Fitness Explosion has granted me honorary core-member status.

In addition to participating in the organizational life of Sisters in Shape, I conducted ongoing interviews (both individual and small-group) with approximately a dozen Sisters in Shape core members over the course of five years. In a few instances, I also conducted onetime interviews with general Sisters in Shape participants. These exceptions aside, talking with the same women over an extended period of time (as opposed to continually talking to more and more Sisters in Shape members) allowed for a fuller range of discourse around their experiences with Melanie, with Sisters in Shape, and with issues of embodiment, activism, and spirituality, especially as their attitudes, ideas, enthusiasm, understandings, and expectations changed in accordance with the ways that health and fitness factored in their lives. While *Body Language* draws most heavily on these interviews with the core members, not all core members interviewed are represented in this work; nor are all the women represented here core members. Overall, however, the experiences of the women not represented in *Body Language* are consistent with those quoted and described throughout the book. In addition, the focus of my discussion and analysis on the specific themes of sisterhood, spirituality, self-esteem, strength, black womanhood, health, and bodily change derives from the frequency with which these topics arose in conversations and interviews.

I taped all interviews and transcribed them as thoroughly as possible, approximating each participant's "voice" by maintaining vernacular speech and by noting word emphases, intonations, imitations, gestures, pauses, and laughter. Additionally, I have tried to represent textually the overlapping dialogue that occurs in conversation, specifically the ways in which many voices often interrupt and intersect to make meaning, to move conversation, and to elaborate on ideas.

Body Language depends largely on texts—records of shared conversations, interviews, and discussions—and at times I provide extensive excerpts to convey the rich contexts within which the Sisters in Shape women perform and theorize their own particular collective and individual identities. I also include my own participation in the interviews or make note of my discursive presence in order to remind the reader that these conversations did not always arise spontaneously, that I asked particular questions to elicit the stories and ideas being shared, that even before I sat down to give meaning to these stories, I guided and helped shape the process.

Articulation: Theoretical and Methodological Foundations

Throughout *Body Language* I attempt to convey the multiple ways that the Sisters in Shape women disrupt the hegemonic images and discourses that seek to define them. By focusing on the group's social interventions—their resistance to, and redefinition of, dominant stereotypes and beliefs—I necessarily attend to the discursive underpinnings of their activisms. Within this context, articulation theory provides an especially apt framework for my project. Simultaneously a mode of analysis, an orientation toward writing, and a theory about language, identity, and power, articulation captures the convergence of both our projects: the Sisters in Shape women's forms of resistance and redefinition (disarticulations and rearticulations) and my own analysis and textualization of their identity politics, itself another articulation of the group.

Because I emphasize the Sisters in Shape women's discourses as the site of meaning for my interpretive readings, my own discursive practices necessarily take on a heightened self-consciousness. This awareness guides me away from traditional ethnography, at least as an overarching mode of scholarship. Even after the discursive shift and the turn toward increased self-reflexivity since the mid-1980s, ethnography continues to exist in a field of expectations—expectations that have long overburdened it and have connected it on the deepest levels with an imagined commitment to some sort of extensive cultural translation. In part because such a translation is neither possible nor desirable, I have turned instead to articulation as a method of analysis and writing that foregrounds the discursive project and the social construction at the heart of all ethnographic work.

The very word *articulation* is rich for any ethnographic project concerned with discourse and the body. In its everyday sense and through its long history, *articulation* has been and continues to be a concept of both body and discourse, as is evident in the definitions provided by the *Oxford English Dictionary*: "one of the segments of a jointed body"; "the structure and mechanism whereby two bones, or two parts of the invertebrate skeleton are connected"; "the utterance of the distinct elements of speech; articulate voice." This dual meaning is united in the language of choreography, for instance, where *articulation* refers to precise body movements as part of the specific language of a dance. *Articulation* also refers to the act of joining, and in this sense *articulation* serves as a valuable discursive hinge between the women of Sisters in Shape and me, between my discourse and theirs.

Cultural studies scholars have drawn on these multiple meanings of *articulation* to develop a theory of cultural practices and productions— including identity formations—as implicitly negotiable and contested (e.g., Laclau 1977; Laclau and Mouffe 1985; S. Hall 1985; Grossberg 1996; Slack 1996; Clifford 2001; Nelson 1999). More specifically, articulation theory arose as an intervention into Marxist approaches to culture, which fundamentally linked cultural production to a society's superstructure; instead, theories of articulation contend that cultural meanings exist only in the moment of articulation, the moment when the intended meaning is not just expressed but also joined to an interpretation. This multidimensional understanding of articulation has been defined and theorized in several different ways, most notably by Ernesto Laclau and by Stuart Hall, both of whom bring together the everyday meanings of *articulation* as "enunciation" as well as "joining," thereby prioritizing the discursive over the structural. Indeed, their definitions clearly resonate with each other in focusing on the ways in which new identities emerge out of articulatory practices of linking distinct but not definitive elements (see, e.g., Laclau and Mouffe 1985;[11] S. Hall 1985; and Grossberg 1996); that is, both Laclau and Hall consider how identity categories join and hold together a range of meanings and associations that have a determinative power despite the lack of any inherent connections between such categories and the elements that constitute them. Hall's consideration of the word *black* as an identity label—from its absence in the Jamaica of his childhood to its significance during the British civil rights movement—illustrates the process of articulation through which *black* comes into being as a historical, political, and cultural category. The various meanings articulated with *black* in the United Kingdom are specific to that historical context, and their absence in the Jamaican context during the same period underscores the ideological dimension of articulatory practices (S. Hall [1991] 1997).

The major distinction between Laclau's (and later Laclau and Mouffe's) and Hall's theorizations has to do with the specific nature of the discursive—for Laclau everything is discursive in the sense of being constituted in language, while for Hall the discursive is metaphoric. Thus, in his theorization, the construction of subjects operates like a language insofar as the referent is arbitrary, not real, even if the effects of such constructions—such as black identity—have material and political consequences in the world. Hall's primary critique of Laclau's theory of articulation is that it unintentionally evacuates the political by collapsing the metaphoric underpinnings of the term *discursive* (Grossberg 1996); that is, the metaphoric comparison to language foregrounds the ideological and political work implicit in all articulations—all identities—because it is in the metaphor that the arbitrariness of language's referential system is exposed. If articulation is simply a process by which subjects are constructed through discourse, then the political work of creating and maintaining those conjoinings falls away. Thus, although my project centers on Sisters in Shape's discursive practices, I rely most heavily on Hall's definitions and theorizations of *articulation*, which leave more space for considering the Sisters in Shape women's embodied praxis and material realities alongside their collective discourses.

By grounding the discursive in the metaphoric, Hall clearly establishes *articulation* as both theory and method—theoretically, *articulation* is a way of making sense of categories and identities through a deconstruction of their recombinant elements, while, methodologically, it is a way of analyzing the discursive practices that hold the elements together under particular social, historical, and political contexts. For Hall, articulation theory provides the foundation for his understanding of identity formation precisely because he sees identity as *dependent* on the work of articulation: "The notion that an effective suturing of the subject to a subject-position requires, not only that the subject is 'hailed,' but that the subject invests in that position, means that suturing has to be thought of as an *articulation*, rather than a one-sided process" (Hall 1996: 6). As is the case with language, the work of articulation is largely naturalized, and social intelligibility demands a certain degree of participation in shared meanings, even as individuals may contest and negotiate specific articulations. The theoretical understanding of articulation as metaphor reveals the lack of inherent meaning associated with any identity.

Methodologically, articulation enables an analysis of the political and ideological motivations joining cultural meanings to identities. For my specific purposes of describing and discussing the Sisters in Shape women's contributions to feminist theories of identity and identity politics, articulation provides a powerful explanatory framework for the particular identity constructions at the heart of *Body Language* while also "enabling us to think" and write such a cultural analysis (Hall quoted in Grossberg 1996). In the chapters that follow, I trace the Sisters in Shape women's disarticulations and rearticulations of such concepts as strength, sisterhood, spirituality, caregiving, and what it means to be a black woman.

Further elaborations on some of the theoretical and political implications of Hall's notion of articulation, together with actual applications of the concept, also provide key touchstones for mapping the significance of articulation for cultural studies in the broadest sense. Jennifer Daryl Slack, for instance, highlights the importance of context for

Hall's theorization of rearticulations in particular: "The context is not something *out there, within which practices occur or which influence the development of practices*. Rather, *identities, practices, and effects generally, constitute the very context within which they are practices, identities or effects*" (1996: 125; emphasis in original). Understanding context as process fosters a situated positionality that prohibits both reductionism and essentialism while also encouraging an acknowledgment of one's own location in the production of any particular context. Throughout *Body Language*, I focus on the makings of specific contexts because such contexts encourage the Sisters in Shape women's variable performances of black womanhood at the center of their nuanced rearticulations. While some may see the co-constitutive nature of context and "identities, practices, and effects" as downplaying or disregarding the power of social structure (see, for example, Collins 1998: 269–270),[12] Hall explicitly situates all articulatory practices within the context of power relations (1985: 95). I similarly frame my readings of the Sisters in Shape women's practices of rearticulation and disarticulation within the context of differential power in the contemporary United States and the consequent material constraints on black women's lives as a result of social oppressions such as racism, sexism, and classism.

Slack also extends articulation beyond theory and method and points to the ways in which it might operate on epistemological, political, and strategic levels by focusing attention on structures of knowledge, power, and action (1996: 112). Integrating all of these aspects, James Clifford (2001) reads the multiple articulations (and related rearticulations and disarticulations) that hold together Kanak politics in New Caledonia with global indigenous politics, an emergent Native Pacific, and issues of authority, mobility, independence, and interdependence. His definition has a useful clarity and, like Hall's, reinforces the significance of process: articulation "evokes a deeper sense of the 'political'— productive processes of consensus, exclusion, alliance, and antagonism that are inherent in the transformative life of all societies" (2001: 473).

Attending to the various ways that articulation theory helps reveal the political phenomena capable of transforming society, Diane Nelson's use of articulation to discuss identity formation and identity politics among Maya cultural rights activists in quincentennial Guatemala (1999) helps demonstrate some of the ways articulation as methodology might enrich ethnographic research. Not only does Nelson foreground the role that articulation plays in all identity formations but she also brings articulation to bear on ethnography through her development of Mark Driscoll's term *fluidarity*: "Taking the articulatory notion of identity seriously, along with the relationality of gringa identity, I develop the concept of fluidarity as a practice of necessarily partial knowledge— in both the sense of taking the side of, and of being incomplete, vulnerable, and never completely fixed" (Nelson 1999: 42).[13] Fluidarity speaks, at least in part, to the vexed nature of ethnography, a project with complicated and contradictory desires at its core, a project both dependent on and demanding of many people whom we come to love, people we ultimately write into at least one set of articulations. At the same time, it forces us to locate ourselves within our research and urges us to embrace the necessarily subjective positions from which we also (re)produce our ethnographic subjects.

But fluidarity doesn't just speak to the practical and ethical difficulties of ethnography; rather, it seeks to respond to the problem of interpreting the subjectivity of an "other. As Clifford has pointed out, ethnographic subjects often make demands of the ethnographer, demands that the ethnographer is incapable of satisfying given the enormity of their scope—demands for an entirely different social ordering, for instance.[14] Even when ethnographic subjects are not making explicit demands of us for radical social and cultural change, our analyses and ethnographic stagings are premised on similarly implicit demands that structure the ethnographic encounter as a discursive negotiation (and, of course, as a material and political negotiation in many cases). Understanding ethnography as a process of discursive as well as material and political negotiation underscores the import of thinking through what an ethical interpretation of an "other" subjectivity may look like.

The loose assemblage of different meanings and uses of articulation described here is especially productive for thinking through some of the discursive parallels—and intersections—between the Sisters in Shape women's discourses and my own interpretations. Articulation offers a paradigm for doing and writing ethnography as a deeply political and, I hope, transformative process and project, one that participates in the larger cultural negotiations for visibility and recognition through engagements with dominant epistemes and other structures of power.

What is especially significant for me in thinking through articulation as a specific theoretical, methodological, epistemological, political, and strategic approach to my ethnographic work with Sisters in Shape is the fact that it describes both of our discursive projects. It highlights the fact that *my* ethnographic project relies on *their* discursive work—namely, the Sisters in Shape invocation of a specifically embodied language to articulate, disarticulate, and rearticulate themselves as local theorists making political and epistemological claims that intervene in, disrupt, and call into question a range of dominant articulations as well as feminist theories of gendered and raced bodies.

Articulation in the senses of enunciating and of joining holds our discursive projects together and points to the entangled nature of my commitment to an "other" as well as to an "other" articulation. Through *Body Language*, I hope that the multiple, mutual articulations I write into being offer a productive intertext for the Sisters in Shape women's own self-representations—those produced not for me but for other women in the world, the series of self-articulations that motivate their ongoing discursive and embodied activisms.

Body, Language, and Embodied Subjectivity: Organization of the Book

The widespread appeal of Sisters in Shape both as an organization and as a social movement rests on the group's collective self-construction through a shared set of body practices and a common set of discourses, through the complex interworkings of discourse and embodiment. Highlighting the specific ways in which the two are deeply entrenched in the Sisters in Shape women's production of their subjectivities, while simultaneously attending to the material realities of black women's lives in a racist and sexist culture, Chapter 2, "Experience: Spirituality, Sisterhood, and the Unspeakable," and Chapter 3, "Performance: Negotiating Multiple Black Womanhoods," jointly establish a foundation for understanding how the Sisters in Shape women mediate some of the tensions in feminist theories of identity politics described previously.

Chapter 2 begins by focusing on the process by which the Sisters in Shape women come to understand and explain their individual body experiences and body modifications through the group's prevailing discourses of their collective social body as well as through a constellation of entangled discourses about improved self-esteem, spirituality, and sisterhood. As is the case with identity, feminist theories of experience and subjectivity have been largely polarized, with a view of experience as irreducible and thus foundational for group identity, on the one hand, and a belief in its fundamentally discursive construction—and, thus, its inadequacy as evidence for grounding historical or theoretical claims—on the other. What the Sisters in Shape women suggest through their embodied subjectivities, however, is that experience is constituted through discourse even as it exceeds it.

Consistent with the Sisters in Shape women's experiences as simultaneously discursive and corporeal, the group's articulations of their collective and individual identity positions are likewise constituted in and through discourse as well as in and through their embodied subjectivities. Chapter 3 investigates the ways in which the Sisters in Shape women continually call the stability of a black women's identity into question through their ongoing performances of multiple black womanhoods. Through a nuanced set of discursive practices together with their bodily praxis, the Sisters in Shape women highlight a movement between various understandings of what it means to be a black woman as well as a black woman participating in Sisters in Shape, and, in doing so, they seem to exemplify Judith Butler's early theory of performative identity.[15] In this context, the troubling question for feminist theory (as well as for others trying to theorize identity) has been whether agency exists in Butler's (and other poststructuralists') theories of disciplinary and discursive processes of subjectification and identity—that is, whether individuals can make choices and take actions to create their identities or whether identity is always created for them through discourse. As many have argued, Butler's (1993) theorization of agency as potentially enacted in the failings of citation, in the resistance to and subversion of dominant interpellations, leaves the *individual's* agency in these actions somewhat ambiguous and open to different interpretations.

By performing the everyday ontologies of their interlocking raced and gendered identities, the Sisters in Shape women contribute a useful response to this question of agency. As is particularly evident in three dominant themes that recur in this context—black women and black bodies, black women cooking (for themselves and others), and black women in and out of groups—the Sisters in Shape women both embrace and contest notions of black womanhood while essentially consenting to and reinscribing the existence of this category, both in their discursive performances and in their everyday lived realities as embodied subjects. Chapter 3 thus highlights the importance of the relationship between tradition and innovation for the Sisters in Shape women's production and performance of black womanhood and suggests that the group's productive rearticulations and disarticulations generate a series of repetitions and citations that motivate social change even as such performativity is linked to certain existing notions of black womanhood.

Sisters in Shape's multiple black womanhoods, through which they resist the hegemonic and singular category of *black women* even as they maintain the relevance of this identity category, lead to unique standpoints that demand black women's social recognition and political visibility. In Chapter 4, "New Bodies of Knowledge," I investigate the ways that the Sisters in Shape women's embodied experiences and their identity performances reinvigorate black feminist standpoint theory (and thus standpoint theory more generally) by pushing it beyond its origins in the presumption of a stable black women's identity and set of shared experiences. Chapter 4 centers on the Sisters in Shape women's explicit interventions into dominant explanations of black women's higher body esteem as compared to white women's and builds on the previous two chapters to explore the ways that Sisters in Shape generates a unique black feminist standpoint that resists reinforcing a fixed identity. Standpoint theory has been crucial in challenging hegemonic feminist theories and epistemologies by drawing from a greater diversity of experiences and by developing more nuanced accounts based in intersectional analyses; at the same time, it has been criticized for collapsing diverse experiences into a singular identity position. By bringing together a set of collective experiences based in both discourse and corporeality (discussed in Chapter 2) and an understanding of Sisters in Shape's particular black womanhood as performative and multiple (discussed in Chapter 3), the women of Sisters in Shape recover the promise of standpoint theory for subject formation, political consciousness, feminist epistemology, and social and political change.

More specifically, against the hegemonic assumptions that black women have greater body esteem than do white women because of different cultural standards, I read a range of Sisters in Shape discourses as a complex cultural commentary that both reorients the dominant discourse of black women's higher body valuation and posits alternative ways of understanding self-esteem in relation to race and the body. Chapter 4 foregrounds such interventions in order to highlight the ways that Sisters in Shape's multiple and embodied selves prompt us to reconsider the complex interworkings of "women's experiences" in relation to feminist theory and feminist activisms as well as the relationship of particular standpoints to new epistemologies.

Building on these analyses of the specific ways that the Sisters in Shape women mediate the often vexed relationship between discourse and embodiment at the center of feminist theories of identity, Chapter 5, "Rearticulating Feminist Identity Politics," concludes *Body Language* by addressing the crucial question of whether identity-based claims to social change and social justice are viable modes of political action. While many theorists have argued against identity politics in this context, Wendy Brown (1993) offers one of the most sophisticated critiques based on her understanding of the relationship between identity-based claims to justice and ressentiment. Brown argues that the controlling logic of ressentiment undermines the potential for a truly democratic politics based on identity because it necessarily reinforces an ontology born of injury and injustice; since politicized identity relies on the continuation of such an injury for its very definition, it cannot help but undermine its claims to justice. While Sisters in Shape may at first seem to offer an alternative to ressentiment with the group's emphasis on self-esteem and empowerment, I interrogate its unquestioned use of *self-esteem* as both a concept and a value and suggest that, ironically, discourses of self-esteem seem to undermine the logic of their primary claims much as ressentiment does. In this case, such discourses ultimately disadvantage the women who rely on them because they tend to overemphasize individual responsibility for social problems, thus depoliticizing the effects of institutional inequalities.

At the same time, however, Sisters in Shape's explicit and fundamental identity as a group whose primary practice is exercise, a practice structured by an investment in bodily transformation, also helps recuperate the political potential of collective identity. Implicit in Sisters in Shape's definition through exercise is a future orientation, an infinite becoming predicated on an ever-changing body, an ever-changing sense of health, and thus an ever-changing (corpo)reality. Foregrounding the signal importance of Sisters in Shape's definition through exercise, together with each woman's enduring belief in a body to come, a future body achieved through Sisters in Shape's programs, I suggest that the group's investment in an alternative future challenges us to consider new and different possibilities for identity-based claims to recognition, justice, and social change perhaps closed to more traditional identity groups seeking rights and recognition from the state. Sisters in Shape's future orientation enables what Brown (1993) sees as a potential alternative to ressentiment, an alternative made possible by a return to the moment of desire in the genealogy of group identity formation; thus, desire replaces the more static sense of being with a dynamic becoming. For Brown, *becoming* transforms the nature of identity-based political claims as ontologically rooted in a constitutive wounding, offering instead the possibility of truly political claims based on an alternative future. In this way, Sisters in Shape offers a distinct and compelling perspective as an identity group whose exercise-based future orientation allows for a political identity structured by something other than a wounding, a political identity that closely couples material bodies with political discourses of desire.

Moreover, because Sisters in Shape is literally practiced in and through women's bodies, the group's identity constructions and knowledge productions necessarily foreground the phenomenological as critical to their politics. As Sonia Kruks has argued, such embodied experiences and ways of knowing can inspire a feminist identity politics that accounts for women's differences while also allowing for the possibility of broader coalitional politics based on affective and sensory intersubjectivities, what she calls the "doubling of embodied awareness" (2001: 166). Chapter 5 situates Sisters in Shape within these theoretical contexts in order to draw out the ways in which their mediations of discourse and embodiment prove fundamental to a rearticulation of feminist identity politics.

Through extended ethnographic engagements with the Sisters in Shape women's collective discourses and embodied practices, *Body*

Language revisits some of the questions that continue to insinuate an intimacy between feminist theory and feminist praxis, questions ultimately concerned with identity formation and the viability of feminist identity politics but nestled in the spaces between discourse and subjectivity, between experience and embodiment. In describing and discussing the appeal of Sisters in Shape as a group specifically of and for black women, the Sisters in Shape women point to and participate in a set of theoretical questions delineated by intersecting strands of feminist theory broadly concerned with identity politics: the importance of experience to collective consciousness, political subjectivity, and social change; the relation of discourse and performativity to identity and agency; and the viability of group identities for political and social claims to justice. Motivated by the Sisters in Shape women's own grounded epistemologies and theoretical insights, by the dynamic ways in which their embodied experiences and discursive practices are co-constituted, I take up lingering questions about the possible strengths and certain limitations of feminist identity politics through an exploration of the tensions among and between language, embodiment, and subjectivity, tensions that might yet inspire alternative theories about the possibilities for political action and social change.

2 / Experience

Spirituality, Sisterhood,
and the Unspeakable

Sisters in Shape has been uniquely successful in sustaining black women's engagement with long-term exercise and dietary changes, and a fundamental part of this success has to do with the organization's ability to forge a collective consciousness. While the Sisters in Shape program explicitly focuses on the practical aspects of black women's health and fitness, its simultaneous attention to the broader social and historical forces underlying black women's disproportionately poor health indicators offers a compelling framework for the Sisters in Shape women's interpretation of their experiences. Although the idea of consciousness raising may evoke stereotypes of 1970s-era feminist talking circles and self-help gynecological explorations, its basic tenets are critical for any group's self-definition and self-determination. Without coming to collective consciousness, groups cannot articulate and rearticulate their multiple and intersecting social positionings in politicized ways, and as Patricia Hill Collins points out, this means they also undermine the possibility of generating critical social theory (1998: xvii).

For Sisters in Shape, consciousness raising is not a particular process or explicit method; rather, it occurs in everyday conversation and in more formal organizational discourse as the women of Sisters in Shape articulate and then rearticulate themselves as black women with the goals of questioning and defying the health status that their race and gender predict. This ongoing articulation of their collective consciousness—the politicization of their personal experiences—implicitly holds Sisters in Shape together as a self-proclaimed group for black women, a group capable of attracting and sustaining black women's interest in a lifelong health and fitness program. The process by which the Sisters in Shape women come to consciousness also reinvigorates questions about the role of experience in social change projects based on identity politics, particularly in terms of the tensions between discourse and embodiment as the principal foundations of experience.

The role of experience in shaping and anchoring social theories has been highly contested within feminist theory. On the one hand, appeals to epistemological, sociological, and historical intervention and to social and political recognition have been staked on an irreducible "women's experience," which is frequently located in the body and thus at least partially resists the oppressive articulations of a phallocentric language and perspective. On the other hand, as Joan Scott argued in her influential 1991 essay "The Evidence of Experience," experience is only ever constituted through discourse and thus calls into question historians' tendency to treat it as a foundational category. For Scott, experience cannot—on its own—carry the evidentiary weight of historical knowledge and critical theory; instead, she advocates for a more historicist approach that assumes the construction and contingency of all experience. In addition, as other critics point out, an overemphasis on the experiential basis of identity also tends to essentialize both individuals and groups in the effort to establish shared experiences.

Attempting to reconcile such polarized positions on the relationship of experience to cultural identity without sliding into the essentialism frequently attributed to identity politics, feminist philosophers like Sonia Kruks (2001) and literary critics like Satya P. Mohanty (1993) argue that the articulation of experience in and through language does not necessarily render it epistemologically suspect. In Kruks's analysis, Scott sets up a "false antithesis" between foundationalism and historicism, and Kruks argues instead that "experience can serve as both a point of origin for an explanation and as the object of an explanation," adding that interpretation and knowledge production can result from either explanation or experience—or both—depending on the context and/or goals of one's research (2001: 138). Kruks uses the example of alternative meanings of the "experience" of domestic violence to make her point: from a historicist perspective, the "experience of being subject to domestic violence" (2001: 138) is constituted by relatively recent discourses on gender, family, violence, and criminality (i.e., experience as the object of explanation), while from a more directly political perspective, women's accounts of their experiences of domestic violence provide the foundations on which to empower women and to develop support programs and legal policies (i.e., experience as the explanatory point of origin).

Mohanty anticipates this point in his theorization of the "epistemic status of cultural identity" (1993). By emphasizing the cognitive nature of experiences for identity in particular—that is, the ways that experiences are always subjected to critical assessment, reinterpretation, and reevaluation within both individual and social contexts—he, like Kruks, foregrounds the fact that experiences can "serve as sources of objective knowledge or socially produced mystification" (51). For both Kruks and Mohanty, attending to the processes by which experiences are socially and discursively constructed enables a historicist approach to the production of cultural identity while acknowledging the foundational effects of experience.

In addition, the process of critical assessment gives rise to an understanding of experience as a type of theory that conjoins individual emotions and interiority with institutionalized social arrangements and hierarchies, and Mohanty draws out the particular significance of such a paradigm for social theories that contest hegemonic representations: "In the case of social phenomena like sexism and racism, whose distorted representation benefits the powerful and the established groups and institutions, an attempt at an objective explanation is necessarily continuous with oppositional political struggles" (51–52). Within this context, the question of whether experience is itself a source of knowledge prior to or outside its discursive articulation becomes irrelevant for Mohanty, who grants the fact of its social construction in order to underscore the importance of such mediation to the production of knowledge and identity. Drawing on Naomi Scheman's work on anger and feminist consciousness raising, Mohanty highlights the intertwined ways that personal experiences are deeply entangled in a complex nexus of individual, collective, social, and political meanings: "Our deepest personal experiences are socially constructed, mediated by visions and values that are 'political' in nature, that *refer* outward to the world beyond the individual" (1993: 46; emphasis in the original). Mohanty's understanding of experience as necessarily imbricated in external social and political constructions resonates with Kruks's point that "practice-based experiences" are intimately connected to "a broader epistemological universe and political agenda" (Kruks 2001: 112), and both theorists underscore the political effects that personal interpretations of experience have on the process of individual and collective identity constructions, even when constituted and constrained by social discourses.

Through such interventions, Kruks and Mohanty reclaim experience from its suspect status as foundationalist knowledge even as they implicitly echo Scott's historicist exhortation to pay particular attention to questions of how experience gets defined as such, how certain experiences become more relevant than others, and how these processes contribute to group accounts of experience that constitute subjects in various fields of power. Throughout this chapter, I draw on Kruks's and Mohanty's work and attend to the ways that the primacy of experience is narrated and shaped by (and within) the group's dominant discourses. Thus, the first part of the chapter focuses on the Sisters in Shape women's descriptions of their personal experiences with the group in order to map the discursive underpinnings of Sisters in Shape's collective consciousness and to highlight the cultural and historical resonances that structure the group's politicization. Close attention to the group's dominant discourses helps locate the Sisters in Shape women in historical and contemporary fields of power, lending insight into the closely affiliated processes of consciousness raising and identity formation. Repeated references to the interlocking themes of improved self-esteem, spirituality, and sisterhood make clear the ways that the Sisters in Shape women's accounts of their experiences together with the group's broader collective discourses are mutually constitutive; together, they demonstrate how the women's individual experiences become understood and named according to the group's dominant idioms even as such personal experiences simultaneously contribute to Sisters in Shape's collective identity.

Perhaps more than anything else, the Sisters in Shape women's accounts of their experiences cohere around the belief that the group achieves its success by helping black women increase their self-esteem. The idea that Sisters in Shape "gives them the strength" to make substantial and lasting changes to their overall health through exercise and alternative ways of eating is critical to their individual and collective experiences and thus permeates the organizational discourse as well as the women's everyday conversations. As with discourses of spirituality and sisterhood, discourses of improved self-esteem contribute to the experiential foundation on which the group establishes its collective identity, and the following two chapters address the ways that the Sisters in Shape women continually return to the topic of self-esteem in their rearticulations and activisms. Given the signal importance of self-esteem to the group's collective identity, it is no surprise that both the value and validity of *self-esteem* are taken for granted throughout the group's discourses, and I defer to their use and valuation of the term in the following chapters, where I take up the Sisters in Shape women's discourses of self-esteem more fully; however, in Chapter 5, I critically interrogate the term within the context of their identity politics.

The Sisters in Shape women also characterize their experiences through the idioms of spirituality and sisterhood, and these deeply interconnected tropes index the ways that this group of black women has been produced in fields of historical and contemporary power relations even as they extend and revise those fields for their own purposes. The extensive role that spirituality plays in the Sisters in Shape women's discourses and in their beliefs about the group's influences on their overall health resonates with black women's long-standing relationships to organized religion and to unofficial spiritual practices (e.g., Frederick 2003; Mattis 1995; Littlejohn 1994; Cannon 1988; Chirea 2003; Grant 1984, [1979] 1995a 1995b; Murray 1979; and McKay 1989). Moreover, black women have a long legacy of drawing on religion and spirituality as key resources in their resistance to oppression and violence and in their community organizing, political reform work, and health activism (e.g., S. Smith 1995; Collins 1991; Joan Martin 1978; Riggs 1994; Townes 1995, 1998; Duggan 2000; Baker-Fletcher 1998; and West 1999); similarly, black women's spirituality and religiosity have been positively correlated with black women's self-esteem and mental well-being (e.g., Littlejohn 1994; Mattis 1995; and Eugene 1995).

Black women's spiritual traditions of resistance and mutual empowerment are frequently upheld as exemplars of what Katie Cannon terms "black womanist ethics" (1988), an orientation toward religion and spirituality rooted in Alice Walker's definition of "womanist" (1983). For Walker, *womanist* builds on the black vernacular term *womanish*— "usually referring to outrageous, audacious, courageous, or *willful* behavior" (1983: xi)—to offer another perspective on feminism, one that allows black feminists and feminists of color to challenge and expand mainstream feminist ideas and theories. Walker's definition of *womanist* first appears as an epigraph in her book *In Search of Our Mothers' Gardens*, a collection of essays that foregrounds the historical and ongoing significance of black women's spirituality in their resistance to wide-ranging oppressions and in their everyday artistic and creative acts; since then, *womanist* has anchored an intellectual movement in religious studies scholarship first introduced by Cannon's *Black Womanist Ethics*. Although womanism is frequently in tension with black feminism (e.g., Collins 1996; Coleman 2006; Cannon 2006; Majeed 2006; Mitchem 2006; Monroe 2006; Razak 2006; Skye 2006; and West 2006), and this project addresses specific debates within feminist identity politics, womanism provides an important touchstone for understanding the Sisters in Shape women's spirituality and their sisterhood as mutually constitutive. More specifically, womanism foregrounds the mutual empowerment that black women have created through their informal spiritual practices, which often operate within the contexts of more formal, patriarchal religions but encourage women to embrace their own and each other's value and worth nonetheless. The Sisters in Shape women are always already positioned within these social and historical fields, and they draw on the language, metaphors, and ideology of spirituality and religiosity to frame their experiences, to understand and uphold their bodily practices, to critique dominant notions of health and wellness, and to posit a particular Sisters in Shape identity.

At the same time, the Sisters in Shape women largely redefine spirituality through discourses of sisterhood, a significant feature of their collective identity as exemplified by the group's very name. And, as with so many Sisters in Shape discourses and experiences, sisterhood is not just taken for granted but rather given a specific Sisters in Shape definition. That is, the Sisters in Shape women implicitly revise overly romantic notions of black women's community as a utopian space of collective strength and resistance by showing some of the ways that black women can be what Melanie terms "ultracompetitive," self-interested, and ready to sabotage another black woman's efforts at self-improvement and success. Against such portrayals of other black women and black women's groups, the overarching Sisters in Shape experience is figured through an exemplary model of sisterhood that the women contend is made possible by virtue of Melanie's charismatic leadership, the positive effects of that leadership on their self-esteem, and the ways that such self-confidence allows them to reach out to and forge relationships with each other. In turn, this particular sisterhood is an important source of spirituality for many of the Sisters in Shape women. Taken together, these tropes not only define Sisters in Shape as a collective group but also provide a language through which the group members come to know their experiences, which they subsequently articulate in a co-constitutive process of individual and collective identity making.

What the Sisters in Shape women make especially clear through these accounts, however, is that experience not only is constituted through discourse but also exceeds it. In this sense, they push us beyond Mohanty's "epistemic status of cultural identity" (1993) and reconciliation of experience to identity, and instead encourage us to consider a broader alliance of discursively constituted experience and embodied, unarticulated experience in the production of collective identity. This is perhaps Sisters in Shape's greatest intervention into feminist theories of experience, subjectivity, and politicized identity. Thus, in the latter part of the chapter I also draw out the ways that the dominant Sisters in Shape discourses of improved self-esteem, spirituality, and sisterhood are intimately tied to experiences of the body in order to emphasize the Sisters in Shape women's reliance on certain knowledge that exists *in* the body, what Kruks calls "sentient knowing, arising from perception, touch, and other sensory experiences" (2001: 33).[1] Through such a corporeal knowledge, the Sisters in Shape women recuperate the phenomenological as critical to questions of the relationship between experience and identity. While sensory knowing largely escapes articulation and is therefore difficult to identify, I read several moments of "unspeakability" in my interviews with the Sisters in Shape women to locate instances where their experiences seem to be extradiscursive. Ultimately, the Sisters in Shape women suggest that, together, the discursive and the phenomenological bases of experience may open up options for an alternative feminist subjectivity and thus a potentially powerful identity politics.

The Spiritual in the Everyday: Foundations of Sisters in Shape

For the Sisters in Shape women, foundational discourses of spirituality determine and shape experiences insofar as they reference and reiterate everyday bodily practices. Within this context, seemingly mundane health activities such as eating properly, going to the gym, and increasing one's exercise intensity level are infused with divine purpose—motivated, in some cases, by God's will—such that the spiritual in the everyday reinforces Sisters in Shape's collective identity through even the most quotidian conversation and dialogue. For example, with her frequent references to divine inspiration, Miriam illustrates the ways that spirituality is operationalized in the daily practice of Sisters in Shape. As one of the group's first members, Miriam is a regular presence in almost all of the Sisters in Shape classes and at all of the group's public events. A dental hygienist in her early 50s, single, with no children, Miriam lives with one of her brothers and his family, and she seems to spend most of her free time with Sisters in Shape, not only working out but also volunteering for events, helping to organize the annual Health and Fitness Explosion, and encouraging new members by asking them about their eating, offering to teach them aerobics routines, and sharing her own Sisters in Shape story.

For Miriam, spirituality and religiosity are overlapping categories, as is clear in the following excerpt, where her language of spirituality structures the Sisters in Shape philosophy while inspiring her long-term commitment to the organization and its goals. I provide a rather long excerpt because Miriam's comments illustrate the almost complete integration of spirituality and religiosity into the Sisters in Shape discourses, an integration that suggests a profound conceptual articulation and not just a discursive overlap. This particular conversation arose several years into my fieldwork, when I already knew Miriam quite well; as we sat down to talk, Miriam asked if she could begin by making a statement:

> I just want to, again, just give Melanie all the credit in doin' what she has done for us, um, in helpin' us and stimulatin' us and just givin' us the confidence and will to keep on doin' it and, with her supervision, losin' weight, and eating right, and just taking our, our [two-second pause] bullshit, and just her bein' so patient and so, such a good trainer and compassionate. Also, I just wanna say, too, and she, um, talks about that a lot, in terms of just havin' the will, no matter what the struggles in life are givin' us, in whatever we do and go through durin' our course of lives, and that with this, we do have to have will, but before we have will, we need that desire, that burnin' desire, and just prayin' to God to give us that will to eat right, to have the appropriate diet, to—I'm getting all confused in what I want to say—but just to eat the right food, to diet right, and strengthen us in our exercise. So, more or less, we must really just have the faith and that will, but first and the most important is the key, the desire, because if we don't have that desire, we won't have that will, that power to eat the right food and exercise and we do need God's help, so all of us just havin' that faith, and put all those, those key words together, and it's very important.

Miriam begins by acknowledging the work that Melanie does to inspire, stimulate, and educate the Sisters in Shape women, and while Melanie certainly deserves much credit in organizing and overseeing Sisters in Shape, she is also a symbol of the project itself, a bodily incarnation and living example of the Sisters in Shape philosophy. Thus, in Miriam's description of Melanie's reminders—commonly reproduced in Sisters in Shape's discourse—about maintaining the will to undertake these lifestyle changes and challenges, she quickly slips into a discourse on God as the underlying source of strength. In this transition from individual responsibility ("we do have to have will") to religious assistance ("just prayin' to God to give us that will to eat right, to have the appropriate diet"), Miriam creates a model wherein everyday bodily practices are rooted in a deep spirituality. Ultimately, for Miriam, the experience of Sisters in Shape is completely and naturally intertwined with her comments about the group's underlying spirituality in a way that fosters their mutual constitution ("we must really just have the faith and that will, but first and the most important is the key, the desire, because if we don't have that desire, we won't have that will, that power to eat the right food and exercise and we do need God's help, so all of us just havin' that faith"). For Miriam, it isn't clear—nor does it need to be—where the individual ends and God begins in terms of practicing the Sisters in Shape way of life. What is significant is the thorough complementarity, even confusion, of the two such that spirituality is operationalized, perhaps even naturalized, in her experiences of Sisters in Shape and, thus, in her understanding of the group's collective identity.

The commitment to the spiritual side of black women's health is often cited as one of the most powerful aspects of Sisters in Shape and one of the features that most clearly distinguishes it from other groups. Many of the women I interviewed claimed that they were initially drawn to Sisters in Shape because spirituality figures so prominently in the group's mission, a fact highlighted in the personal testimonials that constitute the group's collective self-identity. As an example, Toni's description of her initial attraction to Sisters in Shape captures beautifully the personal and political import of spirituality in the group's formative experiences. Unlike most of the Sisters in Shape women I interviewed, Toni, a school counselor in her late 30s, was shy and quiet, pensive, and even a bit reluctant in the few interviews and conversations we had. I was never sure whether I made her uncomfortable, whether she always tended to be reserved, or whether the recent death of her mother and what she described as her ensuing depression made her especially quiet. Probably it was some combination of the three, and other factors we may never have discussed. Regardless, Toni was consistently able and willing to focus on the ways that institutional forms of racism and long legacies of oppression took a toll on black women's bodies and black women's health.

Toni begins her narrative of joining Sisters in Shape by explaining that the group's emphasis on spirituality really drew her to the group: "But the real thing that really caught my eye was the fact that when they talked about, uh, havin' Sisters in Shape, it was not only about physical fitness but it was about spirituality. Spirituality is what captured me because I needed something to fill the void after losin' my mother." Here, Toni's attraction to the spiritual in Sisters in Shape is largely personal, something to "keep [her] goin'" so that she could cope with her mother's death. In this way, Toni's appreciation of Sisters in Shape's attention to the spiritual echoes several of the other women's descriptions of the individual ways that their experiences are articulated through the idiom of spirituality.

A bit later in our conversation, however, Toni quickly politicizes the personal as she elaborates on the intersection of Sisters in Shape, spirituality, and black women's health. At this point, she reiterates the spiritual as a personal draw by repeating the phrase she used to describe this connection in her initial comments—"the thing that caught my eye was spirituality"—but instead of detailing her personal reasons for this attraction as she does in the first instance, she transitions to a much broader discussion of black women's health as defined by Sisters in Shape: "That was one of the things, like I said, once again, the thing that caught my eye was spirituality, okay? Because I said, 'Hey, okay, they're not just focused on health, you look good, you're a size 8.' It wasn't about that; it was about your spirit." Toni contrasts the spiritual with dominant definitions of health in order to critique mainstream tendencies to overemphasize physical appearance in assessing and defining health, a critique that she carries even further by describing inner health, which cannot be determined by physical size: "'Cause if you don't feel good about yourself and let's say you're a size 8 and to some people you look good, it's not gonna last." Toni lauds Sisters in Shape's attention to "mind, body, and soul," and in doing so, redefines health holistically: "So I think that spiritually, that spirituality piece is really great 'cause that person knows that I need to have my health issues addressed, I need to feel healthy." Clearly, for Toni, health cannot be separated from the spiritual, and feeling healthy depends on spiritual health as much as physical and emotional health. Furthermore, as Toni implies, such a redefinition is of dire importance, especially for black women, who are less likely to have body types that align with white heteronormative representations of health and who, consequently, may never consider the ways that they could be living healthier lives.

In this context, Toni also positions Sisters in Shape's spiritual focus on health as a politicized response to gyms where many black women, especially larger black women, feel out of place, uncomfortable, and/or isolated: "It's not like, okay, you have to get to a size 10 and then you can come to our class and take step aerobics. No, you come at the size you are and we work with you from where you are at, you know, and you go from there. So, I, I like the fact that we stress spirituality." Toni's conflating Sisters in Shape's inclusiveness with its emphasis on spirituality highlights the process by which spiritual experiences are produced and sustained through the most quotidian practices and attitudes. For Toni, being "fit spiritually" is crucial to being fit and healthy overall, and a fundamental part of spiritual fitness derives from community, from seeing other black women trying to live healthier lives, from participating in a supportive and encouraging environment: "When I come into the gym, I like the fact that I see a lot of African American women starting to come. And they're all different shapes, and the thing that's real encouragin' is to see someone that maybe weighs about 225 pounds come in here three times a week doin' cardio, doin' weight trainin', and sayin', 'Hey, you know, this is what I had to eat today,' and it's a healthy diet."

This ability to accept other black women regardless of their size and shape, to draw inspiration from their struggles, to develop community with them, brings to life the womanist ethics implicit in the Sisters in Shape philosophy—the emotional well-being and sense of agency, perhaps born of an empowerment fostered by a collective acknowledgment of each other's inherent value and humanity—and enables the women to connect with each other without judgment or competition. Thus, as Toni redefines health explicitly to include the spiritual, she also builds on the emotional and the physical in a way that reveals their deep integration and inseparability, a cornerstone of the Sisters in Shape sisterhood, philosophy, and collective identity.

Melanie's "Ministry"

The significance of a black womanist ethics to the group's processes of collective identity formation is particularly evident in the women's descriptions of Melanie's leadership and their relationships to her as a charismatic leader. The following two examples illustrate how the Sisters in Shape women experience both Melanie and the group in religious terms. In one of my conversations with Miriam, she shared with me her belief that everyone's life involves some sort of spiritual or religious figure—"We always have some kind of inspiration, some angel that's a figure, a image"—and that she understood Melanie to have assumed that status in her own life. At the same time, however, Miriam was also careful to maintain the more formal religious hierarchy, to attribute the profound role that Melanie plays in her life to God's divine intervention: "Thank God, for just leading me to Melanie's direction." For Miriam, both Melanie and Sisters in Shape are made spiritual by the fact that God has led her to them, and through this connection and her positioning of Melanie as an "angel," Sisters in Shape becomes a source of spirituality and the focal point of her life: "My life, for me, is centered around Sisters in Shape and spirituality." Ultimately, Sisters in Shape's spirituality and Melanie's figuration as a charismatic leader provide the generalized support for Miriam's lifestyle changes.

In the more extensive example drawn from the excerpt that follows, Miriam's religious characterization of Melanie and Sisters in Shape is echoed by Cassandra, who more explicitly hails Melanie as a charismatic leader. Cassandra is a lot like Melanie in many ways, especially because she, too, is someone other people would like to be (I discuss the significance of this shortly). She works as a management consultant and, after getting involved with Sisters in Shape, as a personal trainer and aerobics instructor. In her mid-40s, she has been an exercise and fitness fanatic for decades, and though she never worked in the exercise industry before getting involved with Sisters in Shape, fitness has been a fundamental part of her life since she began lifting weights in her early 20s. Her husband has been a personal trainer for most of that time, and she often encourages her teenage daughter to participate in Sisters in Shape's programs and activities. Smart, fit, and beautiful, Cassandra is energetic beyond compare, generous with her time and spirit, encouraging, dynamic, and funny. My most vivid image of her is from an early Saturday morning, before she had become a part of Sisters in Shape. Already done with her workout and headed out of the gym, she came over to where some of the other Sisters in Shape members and I were waiting for Melanie to arrive. Cassandra greeted each woman by name before proceeding to dole out compliments—"Wow, you lookin' great," and "Look at the way your legs are shapin' up," and "Don't you look beautiful with those braids"—all of which she seemed to mean sincerely. She then asked after children's sports teams, parents' health conditions, personal trials at work. Clearly, she was a Sisters in Shape force long before she was even a member.

I met Cassandra during this time—before she joined Sisters in Shape—and I knew she supported the group and often participated in many of Melanie's exercise classes. To me, it seemed she resisted officially joining the group because she didn't think she needed it in the same way that other women did. Cassandra already had a set workout regimen, a healthy diet and lifestyle, and what most people would consider a great body. Not really concerned with losing weight or changing her shape, Cassandra nonetheless began listening to the Sisters in Shape women as she overheard them talking about their exercise and eating practices, and she too began to incorporate the Sisters in Shape plan into her life. She became so lean, with so much muscle definition, in such a short period of time that several of the personal trainers at the gym thought she must be taking supplements to burn fat. While she found such changes to her body compelling, she says it was really the Sisters in Shape sense of community that ultimately inspired her to join the group. Not long after joining, she was certified as a personal trainer and aerobics instructor, and she now plays an organizational leadership role with Sisters in Shape.

Embedded in a larger conversation about many of the Sisters in Shape women's low body esteem and their tendency to focus all their attention on what they dislike about their bodies as opposed to what they might value, the following excerpt begins as Melanie describes one of her methods for getting women to acknowledge some of the positive attributes of their bodies:

MELANIE: And there was a couple of weeks where I said, "Every client I see, I'm gonna tell them, 'I'm gonna challenge you right now, you will, before you look at that area that needs the most improvement on your body, you point out three different, three other areas that look good, before you go'" [Cassandra: Mel, she got it, she blessed, that's her calling], and they're [Cassan-

dra: That's your mission] like, "Okay, okay," and they started doing it.

CASSANDRA: This is your ministry, Mel.

KATRINA: Mm-hm.

CASSANDRA: People wanna look like Mel physically, I like Mel's spirit. I wish I had that kinda spirit [**Allison:** Yes]. I know why I'm here.

MELANIE: You do [have that kind of spirit].

CASSANDRA: But that's, it's not that I'm prouda that, I'm workin' on that 'cause I don't like being that way, and this is where I'm trying to get it from. Unlike Mel, you know, I got an attitude [laughs]. She's like, "Well, Cassandra, that might not be so bad," but that's what I'm saying, this is her ministry, this is her calling, everybody's got a passion and a calling and a path in life and this is it.

MELANIE: I guess it's mine, yeah.

CASSANDRA: It's like natural for you.

KATRINA: And you have your ways, your sheep, and your flocks.

CASSANDRA: Exactly.

MELANIE: Guardian angels is what I call them.

Cassandra immediately understands the power of Melanie's challenges to the Sisters in Shape women, her means of encouraging them to alter their perceptions of their bodies and their low body esteem by having them identify the parts of their bodies that "look good." As Cassandra makes clear in her side comments, Melanie's ability to recast these women's own self-gaze as a positive one is truly inspired: "Mel, she got it, she blessed, that's her calling," and, to Melanie, "That's your mission." With these comments, Cassandra uses a religious metaphor to reframe Melanie's everyday work practices and calls attention to the profound influence that Melanie has on these women's lives. By characterizing Melanie's work as "her calling," Cassandra also grants Melanie the status of a charismatic leader with a "mission," a point that she further articulates when she proclaims: "This is your ministry, Mel." In this way, Melanie is likened to many other charismatic black leaders, folk preachers, lay ministers, and early black women's health workers who were "called" to their life's work (S. Smith 1995: 120).

The transition from the individual to the group occurs as Cassandra moves discursively from the "calling" and "mission" of Melanie's work to Sisters in Shape as Melanie's "ministry." Not only is Melanie "blessed" in her capacity to undertake this work in a meaningful and influential way, but she can also draw people to her such that they collectively create a "ministry." For Cassandra, the two are so thoroughly intertwined that Melanie's ministry and her calling are the same, both a sort of divinely inspired destiny: "This is her ministry, this is her calling, everybody's got a passion and a calling and a path in life and this is it." Most important, others corroborate Cassandra's descriptions and continue to elaborate on it as Katrina does, fully drawing out the religious metaphor with reference to her followers: "And you have your ways, your sheep, and your flocks."

While Melanie agrees that this is, indeed, her calling, she resists seeing herself as a charismatic or religious leader and responds to the fully elaborated metaphor of ministry and flock by altering the terms such that she is equally inspired and motivated by them: "Guardian angels is what I call them." Here, Melanie graciously inverts the power differential implicit in the idea of the Sisters in Shape women as her "sheep" and her "flock" by designating them her "guardian angels," those who enable and protect her and her work, those whom she needs perhaps more than they need her. In this way, Melanie reinforces Sisters in Shape's groupness—its collective mission and work—and extends the foundation for their particular sisterhood as a source of spirituality central to their being.

Despite Melanie's efforts to position herself *within* the group, her status as a charismatic leader, as someone others want to be, is a significant factor in the group's production of its experiences and, thus, its collective identity. My own characterization of Melanie as "someone others want to be" is inspired by a number of different Sisters in Shape women's passing remarks and their narratives about joining the organization in response to seeing or meeting Melanie. Cassandra makes a similar observation in her previous comment about wanting to emulate Melanie's spirit: "People wanna look like Mel physically, I like Mel's spirit." In the context of the group interview, Cassandra's contention that others want to "look like Mel" is a basic assumption, and the other women present readily agreed with Cassandra's claims. In other interviews, two different women described joining Sisters in Shape after seeing Melanie and feeling as though they had the potential to look like her; more specifically, they never felt that they could ever look like the many white fitness leaders they encountered in their gyms, but Melanie's larger, more muscular body seemed to them like a (corpo)real possibility. Core Sisters in Shape members such as Cassandra and Allison also aspired to be like Melanie in their roles as trainers for Sisters in Shape, combining their desire to have Melanie's body type with their desire to inspire women to make major lifestyle changes.

Aside from being someone others want to look like, Melanie is someone the Sisters in Shape women want to be around. Part of what makes her a successful and charismatic leader is her ability to convey interpersonal intimacy when communicating with individual women. In addition to my general observations of this, many Sisters in Shape members offered examples of these intimacies, little moments that spoke to their special relationships with Melanie: late-night phone calls, unique training rituals and inside jokes, shopping excursions, relationship-information sharing, and requests for advice. These everyday acts of friendship, everyday forms of interaction, cultivate for each woman a sense that Melanie is especially invested in her, especially close to her, caring and supportive beyond the broader context of Sisters in Shape. These acts and intimacies contribute to Melanie's status as a charismatic leader and allow her to draw people to her in the way that successful leaders do. By virtue of Melanie's status as a charismatic and powerful leader, her messages—official as well as unofficial—are taken up, "lived" and "experienced" by the Sisters in Shape women, and passed along to other women (through official and unofficial channels) as experiences attesting to Sisters in Shape's effects on their lives, thus reaffirming Melanie's and the group's messages.

From Competition to Community: Redefining Spirituality through Sisterhood

In recounting the everyday spiritual dimensions of their organization, the Sisters in Shape women tend to express their spirituality and to invoke religion in fairly traditional ways. That is, spirituality corresponds to the soul, to sources of inspiration, in some cases to a divine being such as the Judeo-Christian God; likewise, religious references are all situated within a generic Christianity. At the same time, however, the Sisters in Shape women draw on another type of spirituality that departs significantly from its more conventional meanings, a spirituality that both contributes to and results from their own particular sisterhood.

For the women of Sisters in Shape, sisterly Christian love and their particular expression of black womanist ethics are deeply integrated with their everyday experiences and practices of undertaking major lifestyle changes that sometimes go against the cultural traditions and practices of their families and communities. These values emerge out of the women's collective efforts to achieve similar goals and their ability to support each other and to love each other and themselves in the process. As the following examples demonstrate, the Sisters in Shape women also understand their sisterhood as a source of spirituality that directly affects their personal, social, cultural, and political activisms.

The first example is part of a larger conversation I had with Cassandra. In talking about her general experiences with Sisters in Shape, Cassandra begins by saying, "It's, it's, it's powerful"—almost too powerful for words, as is the case with many other Sisters in Shape women (discussed in more depth shortly). To better define that power, she describes a recent Sisters in Shape photo shoot for *Heart and Soul* magazine as an example of the group's collective energy and mutual support. In particular, she remembers being in the locker room after the photo shoot when another woman came up to her and said, "Wow, you guys have so much energy. What was that whole thing about?" In response, Cassandra told the woman about Sisters in Shape, and the woman continued to remark on their "sisterliness": "You guys really act like sisters. I was here when you were getting ready, like were helpin' each other with makeup, with hair, tyin' on scarves, fix up armbands."

In order to best convey her sense of the Sisters in Shape women's energy and mutual support, Cassandra relies on a nonmember's perspective, thus validating her own description with an outside assessment that seems to lend a sense of objectivity to her claims. Intertwined with this other woman's remarks about Sisters in Shape members' energy and mutual support is Cassandra's own affirmation of the woman's characterization of their acting like "real sisters"—"I mean, we were." Overall, the group's positive energy and mutual support have physical and emotional effects on each of the women. For Cassandra, the energy and support of the group are contagious—in this case, helping her overcome the fatigue she felt from having prepared for a wedding and worked a long day before arriving at the gym for the photo shoot: "When I got there, boom, I was wide awake. I mean, you just get caught, you just getting up in it." For her, such energy grows out of the Sisters in Shape women's particular sisterhood, a bond that ultimately forms the foundation of their individual and collective experiences and their group identity: "So the sisters, that, that's the part of it that drew me, that's the part that's makin' me wanna bring other people into the organization." For Cassandra, this positive energy not only attests to the group's sisterhood but also anchors their spirituality, a point she makes explicit much later in the same conversation when I mention that many of the women have described Sisters in Shape in spiritual terms and ask her what she thinks of that. "I think our spiritualness comes from the positive energy in the group," she says, referring again to the *Heart and Soul* photo shoot.

Later in the same conversation, Cassandra makes explicit the logic that unites Sisters in Shape's positive energy, their sisterhood, and their spirituality: "I think our spiritualness comes from the positive energy in the group and that starts with Mel." Here, again, Melanie is granted the status of charismatic spiritual leader for her ability to generate and to sustain this type of positive energy through her own example as well as through her ways of encouraging further sisterhood and support. Cassandra follows up her own equation between Sisters in Shape's spirituality and the group's positive energy with a specific example of how this positive energy spreads throughout the group as each woman is encouraged to enhance another's self-esteem. Cassandra describes this process almost as a chain reaction, beginning with Melanie's teaching them how to communicate with each other, to appreciate and to validate each other: "I'll say to her, 'Mel, wow, look at Nicole.' [*then imitating Melanie*] 'Did you tell her? Tell Nicole. Don't tell me, tell Nicole.'" For Cassandra, this example circles immediately back to spirituality as she moves discursively from her claim to have told Nicole that she's doing really well directly into her belief that such acts are "where the whole spiritual aspect" exists.

As a final example, Miriam integrates many of Cassandra's points about sisterhood, positive energy, and spirituality to reinforce the importance of Sisters in Shape both as a community and as a source of spirituality in these women's lives as they take on the challenges of making major lifestyle changes:

> This is why we are so united in what we do, because we support each other with our problems and just, just helpin' us to lose weight, we are strong and becomin' strengthened, and the struggle to keep up in doin' Mel's class, and eatin' right, and we see someone that's just not, you know, have that step, that energy in class, we give 'em a helpin' hand, just by motivatin', screamin', you know, doin' something to, to make them energized . . . I do see the spirituality in this, this play, I think this is the most important part that plays in us in our, what do you say it, uh, [*slight pause*] conquest to lose our weight and feel good about ourselves, yes. With this support of Sisters in Shape.

In focusing on the Sisters in Shape women's ability to "support each other with our problems" and their collective work to "lose our weight and feel good about ourselves" as sources of strength and spirituality, Miriam reiterates the ways that Sisters in Shape understands itself as establishing new paradigms for black women's community and for black women's spirituality. For Miriam, imagining Sisters in Shape as an ideal type of sisterhood is critical to black women's self-esteem and health activism in theory and practice.

Sisterhood, as a metaphor for family, is especially pertinent because it seeks to overcome black women's broader cultural isolation and social invisibility. For women like Miriam and Toni, both of whom talk about finding solace in Sisters in Shape after the deaths of their mothers and other members of their families, the group's emphasis on sisterhood and spirituality helps them grapple with a literal loss of family connection, an unmooring that both women describe as pushing them into themselves, away from others, and into depression.[2] For Toni, Sisters in Shape offered precisely what she felt was lacking in the months after her mother's death: "I needed something to fill the void after losin' my mother. I needed something to hold on to and I need somethin' to keep me goin' so that I could feel empowered to even go work out." For Miriam, who experienced both the death of her mother and the murder of her sister in the space of a few months, the Sisters in Shape women respond with the same support that family might provide:

> Sisters in Shape has been there supportively, um, one even came to the service and representing Sisters in Shape, which was, um, [Kim: This was for your sister?] this was for my sister and, um, Charlie, she came, and I knew it was for the support of the sisters. And they also gave me, um, a massage certificate, um, to kinda help to release some of that stress, that tension from all of it, so, yes, exercising and with sisters in help, just bein' there for me is so important.

Here, Miriam's reference to the Sisters in Shape women as "sisters in help" (perhaps a telling slip of the tongue?) captures beautifully the ways she herself understands their sisterhood in both metaphoric and real material terms, a point that Charlie reiterates when she says, "It becomes like your larger family, and it's good. That helps, it helps a lot, not just in here but anything you do."

For many other black women, feelings of isolation undoubtedly also stem from the daily struggles of trying to survive in a racist, sexist, and antifat culture, from the unlikelihood of seeing themselves reflected in media representations or any other number of social mirrors. Both Toni and Sonja praise Sisters in Shape for creating an inclusive social space where black women can be seen and recognized as themselves, a space where they can join with other women who do not make assumptions about their right to be in the gym because of their weight or their race. As Toni points out, with Sisters in Shape "it's not like, okay, you have to get to a size 10 and then you can come to our class and take step aerobics. No, you come at the size you are and we work with you from where you are at." In a related example, Cassandra shares a story about one of her colleagues, a woman whose discomfort and isolation at her New Jersey suburban gym underscore the importance of Sisters in Shape's work in helping women resist these and similar oppressions: "She's going to that strip-mall gym, where she wears these really big clothes, then she looks around, 'I'm the fattest one in there, I'm the only black one in there, uh duh duh duh duh.'"

Such feelings are compounded by these women's sense that other black women are "ultracompetitive," that they will "stab you in the back in a minute." Even Sisters in Shape members like Justine talk about their own participation in this "degrading" behavior before joining Sisters in Shape:

> And I used to look at other women, degrading myself, other women who were heavier, say, "Oh, look at her, she knows she doesn't need to be eating that ice cream," or "She knows she doesn't need," and I mean, I was very degrading to women. Today the way I feel is I walk in the gym, I see a woman on a, on a, I don't care what her weight or her shape, that woman is going to love herself. And I'll do like this [nods], or I'll say like, "How you doin'?" or just like, "Hello," just to give her that encouragement because to me, then we're together, we're in a struggle together understanding that there are lots of things out there to stop us from loving ourselves.

Here, as Justine makes clear, part of the Sisters in Shape philosophy is that increased self-esteem enables women to come together in struggle, and this type of sisterhood—which virtually all the Sisters in Shape women I interviewed mention—resonates with the group because it first calls attention to, and then diminishes, the social isolation and invisibility that continue to oppress black women.

The Critique of Competitive Others

The collective logic by which the Sisters in Shape women come to understand their own sisterhood as a critical source of spirituality— and, in some cases, to redefine spirituality *as* sisterhood—depends in large part on their implicit critique of an overly romanticized representation of black women's community as generated by popular media such as black women's magazines, films such as *Waiting to Exhale,* and academic works that unquestioningly celebrate black women's groups as sites of social resistance.[3] The combination of these sources and similar ones creates a sense of black women's communities as essentially utopian spaces, safe reprieves from external sources of oppression and danger and virtually without internal conflict. While the Sisters in Shape women do not reference specific examples of an overly romanticized sense of black women's community, their repeated references to competition, strife, general negativity, and lack of support among non–Sisters in Shape "black women" help them demarcate the ways that they experience their participation with the group as differing sharply from their participation with other groups of black women, thus reinforcing the importance of sisterhood and/ as spirituality to the group's articulation of its experiences and to its collective identity.

Several Sisters in Shape women offered examples of black women's competition and general inability to support each other, especially in contexts relating to the body and to bodily "improvements," to explain what makes Sisters in Shape unique in their minds. Against these personal narratives detailing instances of black women's lack of community, the Sisters in Shape women describe their own group in religious metaphors to position themselves as a sisterhood and as a primary source of spirituality, an equation that continues black women's long tradition of womanist ethics and the rearticulation of hegemonic religious discourses and practices, their long tradition of drawing on the spiritual for social, cultural, and political critique and resistance. Their understanding of their own sisterhood as an important source of spirituality thus allows them to reimagine black women's power—their power—to alter institutional oppression and to intervene in dominant cultural discourses of black women's health and wellness. At the same time, by redefining spirituality through sisterhood, the Sisters in Shape women imbue their lifestyle choices with a certain cultural authority; that is, if sisterhood is spiritual, then their decisions to attend to each other and to themselves within such a context are not only appropriate but also important ways to dedicate their lives.

Especially prevalent are personal narratives describing competition and lack of support between Sisters in Shape leaders and other black female personal trainers at 12th Street Gym, where Sisters in Shape began. In one conversation, Melanie and Cassandra offered a general overview of some of the backstage politics that occur at the gym between the Sisters in Shape women and other black female personal trainers. The following example involves Angie, a medical doctor and personal trainer at 12th Street Gym who is not affiliated with Sisters in Shape. The conversation was prompted by Melanie and Cassandra's prior discussions of a longtime core Sisters in Shape member who had put herself on a fad diet, something Sisters in Shape strongly discourages. Such extreme dieting contradicts the group's efforts to encourage participants to think of eating as significantly connected to exercising and to healthy living generally; in fact, a central concept of their philosophy is that women should not fear food, as many women do after years of living in a culture saturated with unrealistic, airbrushed representations of women's bodies, constantly changing fad diets, and an ever-increasing range of low-calorie substitute foods. Gossip about this particular Sisters in Shape member's "desperate" attempts to lose weight quickly, as opposed to trusting the long-term and proven nutritional plan that the group has developed, inspired Melanie's anger and Cassandra's sympathy, and Cassandra's attempts to help Melanie contextualize the woman's transgression led to her description of other extreme diets and eating plans used by other, non–Sisters in Shape trainers at the gym.

This is the context in which Cassandra reports that Angie's program of nutritional counseling involves only 300 grams of carbohydrates per day, an amount that both she and Melanie deem far too low for the type of cardiovascular exercise and weight training that the Sisters in Shape women and Angie's clients do. Melanie transitions from a comparison of different perspectives on nutritional counseling, and, especially, the dangers of Angie's recommendations, to the suggestion that Angie's medical degree grants her a certain credibility despite her "giving such wrong information."

MELANIE: They go to her because she's an MD; they feel safe, [Cassandra: Exactly, that's exactly what it is] and what they don't understand is that [Cassandra: That's wrong] she's giving such wrong information.
CASSANDRA: Yup!

MELANIE: It's really sad, it's very sad. And I don't know what she's tryin' to do. But somebody said she's now doin'—I don't know if it was you who told me—lose twenty-two, lose twenty-two pounds in a month.

Claiming, "I don't know what she's tryin' to do" as a rhetorical connection between Angie's "giving such wrong information" and her offer to help people "lose twenty-two pounds in a month," Melanie establishes the foundations of a broader perspective on what she later refers to as Angie's "manipulative" behavior (cited in the following example) and the implicit need to attract clients (a task that can be especially difficult for black female trainers who do not work with Sisters in Shape, since it is the only group explicitly for black women at this particular gym and throughout the greater Philadelphia area).

Within this context, Cassandra details her own ongoing interactions with Angie, who repeatedly asks to take Cassandra's measurements whenever she sees her in the gym and is with one of her clients. Taking measurements is common practice for Sisters in Shape and other weight training programs, as it helps participants evaluate and understand their bodies in terms of body fat percentages and size as opposed to solely their weight.

CASSANDRA: She does keep askin' me if she can do my measurements again.
MELANIE: Why?
CASSANDRA: I dunno. I don't want her to. I don't want any part of anything that she, I mean, I say, "How ya doin', Ange, it's good to see you," but I don't really wanna be associated with that, and she always asks me when she's around her clients because they'll say, "Wow, she's really, she really has low body fat."
KIM: Oh, so they think, so that they'll think that you're her—
MELANIE: She's takin' credit . . . this is why she wants to be your friend, this is why she's running after you, this is why she's talking to you all the time. She's gonna take advantage, she's gonna consider you her product and that is what happened.
CASSANDRA: She never asks me when we're one-on-one, but as soon as she gets around her clients and they pay me a compliment

[**Melanie:** She's a manipulator.] . . . she's, "Oh, Cass, I still have to get your measurements; I still have to get your measurements," and she's showin' off.

. . .

Kim: And she's really takin' advantage of you.
Melanie: She is. She's taking advantage of you.
Cassandra: She is taking advantage of me, she really is, yeah.
Melanie: I knew it, I knew it, I knew it [*with added emphasis*].
Cassandra: Yup, you called it a long time ago.
Melanie: I know her. I know her, Cassandra. I know her . . .
Cassandra: Mel told me she was gonna do that [**Melanie:** I know her like a book.], but I thought maybe Mel didn't know what she was talkin' about. She called it. [**Melanie:** I called it.] Yeah.
Melanie: I'm sorry that it happened that way, though.
Cassandra: Yeah, it's amazing, though, you know.
Kim: There's so much competition.
Cassandra: There is, there is, there is.

As Cassandra and Melanie make explicit, by asking to take Cassandra's measurements at these moments, Angie implies to her clients that Cassandra is also one of her clients and that Angie is responsible for Cassandra's muscular, lean body. In this way, Angie can "take credit" for the work that Cassandra has done; as Cassandra says, Angie is "showin' off" by asking to take her measurements in front of other women.

My own reiteration of their point that Angie is "taking advantage" of Cassandra is quickly elaborated by both Melanie and Cassandra. The conviction in Melanie's statements ("I knew it, I knew it, I knew it" in response to hearing Cassandra recount Angie's attempts to present her as her own client), together with the fact that she anticipated such manipulative behavior (Cassandra's "Mel told me she was gonna do that" and Melanie's "I know her like a book"), moves the conversation to a more general assessment of the backstage politics that surround Sisters in Shape and implies an ongoing struggle for status within the gym, especially given the success and widespread publicity that Sisters in Shape has achieved, not only in that immediate environment but throughout the city and nationally. In the end, I summarize what I hear them saying about these ongoing struggles—"There's so much competition"—which is reiterated by Cassandra's hearty agreement, "There is, there is, there is."

In a similar example, Melanie and Cassandra talk about two interactions with Martha, another black female trainer and competitive bodybuilder at the gym, to illustrate the degree to which these backstage politics erupt in everyday contexts. The topic of Martha is first introduced when Cassandra asks whether Martha has ever been involved with Sisters in Shape, prompting Melanie to describe Martha's generally negative attitude and haughtiness around the gym. Melanie attributes Martha's hostility to rumors that Martha's recent victory at a bodybuilding competition was contested by some of the judges. Since Melanie was a judge at that competition, she believes that Martha thinks she may have been one of those who voted against her. Later in the conversation they return to the subject of Martha, as Melanie tells the story of an incident in which a group of Sisters in Shape women indirectly challenged Martha at a health fair:

> As Sisters in Shape continued to grow and she got more jealous, um, we were at the Health Quest Fair last October and she was there handing out her cards and she was, and the sisters [*laughs*], Miriam was the ringleader, she had about five of the Sisters in Shape, grabbed a bunch of, "Mel, where your cards at?" [*conspiratorially, imitating Miriam*], grabbed a bunch of cards 'cause they saw her handin' out all her cards, and they started runnin' around, and they all had their T-shirts, and they were like, you know, handin' out cards, and she had made a comment to somebody, once somebody overheard her making some kind of or maybe she said it to Charlie [*a Sisters in Shape core member*], "Hmmph, I don't know why people don't wanna share," as if she shoulda been sharing our booth.

Melanie cuts to the core of this issue by framing the incident as one of jealousy resulting from the tension between Martha as an individual trainer and Sisters in Shape as a group practice: "Sisters in Shape continued to grow and she [Martha] got more jealous." The distinction between individual and group is further accentuated in the way the Sisters in Shape women—and not Melanie—deal with Martha and what they perceive to be her encroaching on their physical, business, ideological, and group space: "Miriam was the ringleader, she had about five of the Sisters in Shape, grabbed a bunch of, 'Mel, where your cards at?,' grabbed a bunch of cards 'cause they saw her handin' out all her cards, and they started runnin' around, and they all had their T-shirts." Physically marked as a group with their matching Sisters in Shape T-shirts, this group of "sisters" effectively, if indirectly, sends Martha a message that makes explicit their group status and their collective ownership of Sisters in Shape as their project, not Melanie's individual personal training business. In essence, it is this difference, at least according to the rhetorical arc of Melanie's narrative, that contributes to Sisters in Shape's growth and success as well as to its being a fundamental source of jealousy for some of the other black female trainers who must compete for clients.

After this example, Cassandra offers one of her own to further emphasize Martha's negative behavior and attempts at backhanded criticism. In this case, Martha attempted to engage Cassandra in a dialogue about Sisters in Shape's absence from Sistahs, a large annual event for black women sponsored by one of the local radio stations: "She sat her fire-plug ass out on the bench out there, 'I didn't see Sisters in Shape [at Sistahs], and I thought I heard them say they were gonna be there' [in a huff, imitating Martha]. I didn't even acknowledge it. I don't talk if people are not talkin' to me directly." A bit later, after Melanie exclaims that Sisters in Shape does not owe Martha an explanation since she has nothing to do with the group, especially given Martha's delight in Sisters in Shape's failing to show up at Sistahs, Cassandra describes the situation in more detail: "Right out here [gesturing at a nearby bench], right down here underneath that sign. And waited good till she saw me coming down and goin' to the locker room and hollered it out loud, like I was gonna say, 'Oh, by the way . . . .' Don't pitch me, I'm nobody's stick."

Through her account, Cassandra offers an intimate sketch of the interpersonal politics operating at this gym, and Melanie responds by summarizing the whole affair in succinct and direct terms: "She's just like, she's, she's now on this thing to be ultracompetitive." Though initially cast as an individual experience between Martha and Cassandra, the dialogue that ensues again positions Martha's "thing to be ultracompetitive" as a tension between individual and group, a conflict that emerges when Martha questions Sisters in Shape's absence from Sistahs.

Winding down these descriptions of competition between Sisters in Shape and other black women at the gym, Melanie thematizes the previous, more extensive examples of competition, interpersonal strife, and general backstage politics surrounding Angie's and Martha's exclusion from Sisters in Shape with some direct talk about competition among black women, of which she too is a part.

MELANIE: It could be all that, that, that Angie's camp, Mel's camp, Martha's camp bullshit.

CASSANDRA: Ooooh!

MELANIE: 'Cause I knew it was gonna happen. I know that if I had, that if I didn't let Angie into this circle that it would become this against that against that, and that's exactly how she is to me.

CASSANDRA: Yeah.

MELANIE: I don't care. God will take care of me. 'Cause I'm not into that. Yeah. But I just know. What I thought would happen is coming to be. You got three black women in the house, fightin' each other. That sucks.

Here, Melanie begins by acknowledging her own role in these struggles, first with reference to her "camp" and her keeping Angie from joining Sisters in Shape in a leadership capacity and then with her presumed foreknowledge that excluding Angie would lead to precisely this situation. What Melanie does not articulate in this excerpt, however, are her reasons for not "[letting] Angie into this circle." In one of the early interviews I conducted with Melanie and several of the first Sisters in Shape members, Melanie responded to the women's appreciation of her leadership by pledging that everyone affiliated with Sisters in Shape would always have a similar attitude:

I intend to be very very very selective about who comes aboard on our team and how important [positive energy] is. The people who are gonna be trainin' for Sisters in Shape have to be compassionate. They have to care about people; they have to have good interpersonal skills, they have to have a high level of professionalism, and they just have to care, they have to, they have to provide the same qualities that I'm hearin' that I'm providing. And no ifs, ands, or buts about it. Anybody with negative energy, I will run from them as fast as possible. I always run from negative energy as fast as I can.

While Angie would undoubtedly not characterize herself as having negative energy or lacking compassion and professionalism, Melanie clearly sees her that way when she questions Angie's recommendation that clients eat only 300 grams of carbohydrates a day. In an attempt to develop Sisters in Shape as a positive, supportive group for black women and their health and fitness, Melanie relies on discourses of competition among mostly *other* black women—although she also embodies and sustains that sense of competition through her descriptions of it—in order to convey a Sisters in Shape experience of sisterhood lacking in the broader community of black women.

In calling attention to the qualities necessary for future Sisters in Shape trainers, Melanie seems to attribute competition among the black female trainers associated with the different gym "camps" to narcissism, negative energy, a general lack of compassion toward other women, and an inability to support other women's work toward major lifestyle changes. In so doing, she posits a Sisters in Shape group identity premised on the opposite traits of positive energy and support for other women, traits frequently reiterated by Sisters in Shape members attempting to describe their experiences with a group they perceive to be different from other black women's groups and other groups of black women. For instance, in one interview, two women told me that one of the features that distinguishes Sisters in Shape is the camaraderie that Melanie engenders; when I asked them how she does that, they immediately responded, "Positive energy." One of the women elaborated in language common to many such descriptions: "Everything we do, we meet each other, everything has to come across as positive. We never let anybody or anything inflict any negative energy around us because negative energy has gotten us to the point where we were."

The fact that this woman responded to my question about Melanie's leadership with a collective *we* underscores the extent to which the idea is a part of each woman's experiences with Sisters in Shape as well as a part of the group's self-understanding and self-presentation. While women like Angie and Martha have not been invited to participate in Sisters in Shape as trainers—perhaps the only roles they would accept—they have been invited to join Sisters in Shape as members who might participate in classes, workshops, group events, and other Sisters in Shape programs. Their decisions not to join Sisters in Shape on this level may mean many things, but above all, such decisions seem to suggest that the "Angie's camp, Mel's camp, Martha's camp bullshit" will persist, continually delineating the boundaries that allow the Sisters in Shape women to see themselves as a rare form of sisterhood.

Melanie's final assertion draws on all of these examples to fully intervene in any discourses of black women's community as utopian space: "You got three black women in one house, fightin' each other." Even as she debunks any notion of an all-inclusive, supportive community of black women, she simultaneously embraces the ideal of such a community in her final lament—"That sucks"—and registers her disappointment that no such community exists. That such an ideal does not exist in reality cannot be surprising, especially given the economic, social, cultural, and personal contexts in which these women's experiences are embedded. That is, the idea of a utopian community can only ever be an ideal due to any number of influences and oppressions that collaborate to create conflict, including those perpetuated by the Sisters in Shape members even as they resist others. In these specific cases, the Sisters in Shape women's collective discourses and group actions help undermine overly romanticized notions of black women's collective community, thus establishing the social contexts against which they ironically seek to present themselves as just such an idealized group.

Spirituality and sisterhood are important aspects of Sisters in Shape's collective identity, and therefore critical foundations of the individual women's understandings and articulations of their experiences, precisely because they address and reflect this group of black women's needs in the urban United States today. These interconnected tropes not only delimit Sisters in Shape's boundaries and uphold the group's sense of itself as unique among black women's groups, but they also bring together historically relevant ways of being in the world, ways of acting in and on the world, that simultaneously give meaning to the Sisters in Shape women's individual experiences. As we have seen, nestled within and among these narrative accounts of individual women's experiences with Sisters in Shape are other narratives and discourses that help determine and sustain them: the historical, cultural, and group articulations that lend insight into the specific logics of these particular productions and reproductions of experience and identity.

Identity, Embodiment, and Extradiscursive Experiences

The entangled discourses that help the Sisters in Shape women interpret and articulate their experiences within a broader social and political context are intimately related to their embodied practices. Sisters in Shape is, after all, fundamentally about the body. As mentioned earlier, the Sisters in Shape women intervene in feminist debates about the importance of experience to collective identity, identity politics, and social change by highlighting the ways that experience is always discursively constituted while simultaneously extradiscursive. Though it is difficult to capture and convey experiences that exceed articulation, the Sisters in Shape women offer glimpses of such experiences in the moments when language fails them; when experience is unspeakable; when confused utterances, placeholders, and simple sounds stand in for more standard modes of articulation. In these moments—inspired by both spiritual awe and physical sensations—the Sisters in Shape women prompt a reconsideration of the enduring, but false, binary between experience as discursively constructed and experience as largely independent of our language for describing it, an ongoing tension that has sidetracked important questions for feminist theory and feminist identity politics.

Within this context, Sonia Kruks draws attention to what she sees as the limits of discourse analysis for explaining the specific processes through which demands for recognition inspire collective action. While maintaining the value of discourse analysis for mapping the "discursive spaces in which it has become possible for narratives of women's oppression and demands for recognition to emerge" (2001: 132), Kruks argues that feminist theory must "hold onto the concept of experience and must attend to the ways in which experience can exceed discursivity" (133) if it is to account for the impetus to political practice. Drawing on Merleau-Ponty's phenomenological description of the body-subject, Kruks assumes a knowledge in the body—"ways in which we come to know, think, and act with our bodies" (144)—as key to locating extra-discursive experience. More specifically for feminist theory and politics, she argues that the affective nature of embodied subjectivity, the feelings and emotions that lie beyond both the postmodernist and the rationalist conceptualizations of the discursive, inspires feminist identification, practice, and action. Kruks's theorization of the affective underpinnings of feminist praxis offers insight into the political and oppositional significance of the Sisters in Shape women's articulation of their collective identity through experiences that derive from both affective embodiment and collective discourse even as those experiences are simultaneously structured by the individual and collective understandings of them. Within this context, I offer here several examples of the Sisters in Shape women's moments of unspeakability in order to outline the full process—together with discourse—through which the Sisters in Shape women generate a politicized identity that not only resonates with large numbers of black women but also moves them to action.

Consistent with the dominant Sisters in Shape discourses that constitute and constrain individual experiences and contribute to the group's collective identity, the following examples of "unspeakable experiences" likewise emerged in discussions of improved self-esteem, spirituality, and sisterhood. Unlike many of the examples recounted earlier in this chapter, however, the contextual themes recede to the background as these different Sisters in Shape women attempt to convey the embodied feelings at the center of their experiences with the group. Thus, these examples call attention to the failures of language and the subsequent demarcation of blank space as ways of highlighting the extradiscursive aspects of Sisters in Shape experiences.

In one of our earliest interviews, Miriam weaves many familiar Sisters in Shape themes together with her beliefs about how the group has affected her spiritually:

> When I first started, um, I still lacked, a lack of self-esteem, confidence and stuff. I've always been a spiritual person, but

this has like, uh, been extreme, higher with me, the company of friends, the priorities, always gonna be workin' out. It's like, it's gonna be a lifelong thing for me, anything that I can do for Sisters in Shape, I'm going to do it 'cause, I don't know, it has inspired me in that words can't say [*trails off into two-second pause*]. And spiritually, it's been so motivating to me that I just feel so, so overwhelmed.

Though thoroughly integrated into her account of how her experiences with Sisters in Shape have increased her self-esteem and her spirituality, Miriam's feelings about spirituality and Sisters in Shape remain largely unspeakable—"it has inspired me in that words can't say" and "spiritually, it's been so motivating to me that I just feel so, so overwhelmed." What may at first sound like confusion in Miriam's claim, "I don't know . . . words can't say," takes on a more profound meaning in the longer, two-second pause that follows, a pause in which she may be considering which words could suffice before she simply allows the thought to trail off, deciding instead to let her feelings and experiences escape the confines of an inadequate language. Similarly, when following up with a seemingly more concrete point about Sisters in Shape's underlying spirituality and inspiration in her life, Miriam never actually conveys or even describes her feelings except to say that she is overwhelmed by the experience, by what she knows but cannot find the language to communicate. Rather than continue trying to translate her feelings and her experiences into metaphor or tangible example, Miriam permits the sense of being overwhelmed to stand on its own, a way of letting her feelings supersede the discursive. Here, then, Miriam's unwillingness to speak the spiritual, to render comprehensible her affective and embodied sense of it and of Sisters in Shape as a mode of spirituality, together with her inability to do so, attests to the ways that her experiences with the group clearly exist in deeply embodied sensibilities that exceed and resist discourse.

In a similar example, Justine offers a Christian parable to describe the effect that Sisters in Shape and Melanie have had on her life. Echoing many of the themes evoked by other Sisters in Shape members, Justine's invocation of unspeakability likewise indexes the importance of both the idea (discursive understanding) and the sense (extradiscursive knowledge) of Sisters in Shape as a profound experience—a feeling that in turn contributes to the group's collective identity formation. In her early 30s, Justine has had an on-again/off-again relationship with Sisters in Shape, though an unplanned pregnancy and the family and relationship crises it provoked most likely account for her initial withdrawal from the group. When I first met Justine, she had recently completed her master's degree in educational psychology and was just beginning her first job. She was ecstatic about life, and everything seemed full of promise to her, especially her recent commitment to Sisters in Shape. During that first interview, she told me that Sisters in Shape had helped remind her what it really meant to understand the body as a temple, another example of spiritual discourse woven into the everyday language of the group. Justine was on a newfound "mission" to cleanse her body, to "purify her temple," and she had sworn to maintain its "sanctity" in the future.

Clearly intelligent and articulate, Justine immediately pointed out the innumerable ways that black women and their bodies are rendered invisible in our culture. She saw Sisters in Shape as a way of teaching women to honor their bodies as sacred spaces, a new way of thinking about themselves and their bodies that might intervene in their social erasure. I thoroughly enjoyed talking with Justine each time we met and was both surprised and disappointed when I learned that she had left Sisters in Shape. The next time I spoke with her, she was about seven months pregnant—round and glowing—and had been back with Sisters in Shape for a few weeks. In this context, Justine used the biblical parable of Christ encouraging Peter to walk on water to frame her recent experiences and her return to Sisters in Shape.

She prefaced her telling of the parable by updating me on her situation, discussing the factors that motivated her to return to Sisters in Shape and recounting how she felt during her first meeting with Melanie after her six-month absence. Knowing that getting in shape and being around the other Sisters in Shape women is "what works for me," Justine decided to talk to Melanie about a workout routine that she could do during the rest of her pregnancy. She describes the importance of that conversation to her renewed commitment to herself: "I sat with her one day, and I cannot tell you, it was like I was on a high, and all I did was discuss what was goin' on with me and my need and my understanding that I needed to be back in here." In talking about her need to make "that commitment to myself again," Justine recounts a lesson she recently heard at church:

> I went to this sermon, um, they were talking about Jesus, and Jesus was standing on the water, and Peter is in the boat and he's going to, he's like, "Well, Lord, if it's true that I can walk on water, then let me walk towards you," and so he gets out on the water and he keeps walking towards Jesus and takes his focus off of Jesus and he falls into the water. And I saw myself as Peter, that I was takin' my focus off the things that were more important, the things that help me feel good about where I was, and I started setting boundaries. When I talked to Melanie that day, I can tell you, right after that—and I'm not saying Melanie's God or anything—I'm just saying, just knowing what she's about, that the whole piece matters, the physical, the emotional, and the spiritual matter.

Justine conveys her description of this meeting with Melanie and her decision to return to Sisters in Shape in language similar to that of Miriam's unspeakability: "I sat with her one day, and *I cannot tell you*, it was like I was on a high" (my emphasis). For Justine, memories of her participation with Sisters in Shape, along with her anticipation of future participation, are enough to put her "on a high," which she seeks to articulate but ends up summarizing with the phrase "I cannot tell you." While the phrase "I cannot tell you" may be a shorthand placeholder for something that could be articulated but at much greater length, I want to suggest instead that the phrase stands in for that which is impossible fully to capture and convey, in this case the particularly embodied quality of the "high" that Justine experiences after her meeting with Melanie.

The parable of Jesus coaching Peter to walk on water becomes Justine's way of translating into language what she had earlier been unable to describe; she contextualizes the parable by reading herself into it as Peter. Following her use of this religious reference, Justine's "I cannot tell you" becomes "I can tell you" as the parable makes concrete that for which she had previously failed to find language. That is, the parable is key in helping Justine structure her understanding of her participation with Sisters in Shape and the role that Sisters in Shape plays in her conceptualization of her health as an integrated whole: "When I talked to Melanie that day, *I can tell you,* right after that . . . just knowing what she's about, that the whole piece matters" (my emphasis). Whereas Justine's "I cannot tell you" refers to an embodied and emotional feeling (a "high"), her transition to "I can tell you" is paralleled by a transition to a much more nameable idea, the idea that focus and holism are fundamental to her health. This distinction between the types of knowledge indexed by the two phrases further underscores the frequently extra-discursive quality of embodied sensibility even as such experiences are always also entangled with the discursively constituted and constrained experiences at the center of identity formation.

In an example that has less to do with spirituality and more to do with the embodied sensations at the heart of the Sisters in Shape experience, Cassandra relies on sounds of exultation to convey how Sisters in Shape makes her feel about/in/as her body: "You know what's more important to me than how I look? How I feel . . . Whooo! I love the feel. I feel good . . . that feelin', you know, that's the thing." In trying to capture how Sisters in Shape makes her body feel, Cassandra never actually describes the feeling (aside from the generic "good"), despite her repeated references to the feeling itself; rather, she expresses the feeling through her "Whooo," a sound that many of the other Sisters in Shape women used to express the embodied joy and exhilaration of their experiences in Melanie's aerobics classes. Given this common practice, Cassandra simply assumes that her exuberant "Whooo" is something others can understand and relate to ("that feelin', you know").

The difficulty of finding the words to adequately describe Sisters in Shape as a source of spirituality and/or embodied experience is not an uncommon problem. Spiritual awareness, feelings, and bodily sensations are often just beyond the reach of language. This is not to suggest that spirituality and embodiment exist before or entirely outside language, however; although we may not have a precise language for expressing feelings associated with spirituality or with our bodies, at least some of our experiences of them are always already shaped by the discourses in which we are produced and reproduced as subjects, including the discourses contending that such experiences are beyond articulation. At the same time, some aspects of spirituality and embodiment may also escape the totality of language.[4] Regardless of the social determinants of gender and race, for instance, Miriam, Justine, and Cassandra all feel and thus come to know many of their Sisters in Shape experiences through their bodies in extradiscursive ways, and through the acts of trying—and failing—to speak their embodied experiences, they highlight the inseparability of discourse and embodiment as sources of experience and, ultimately, collective identity.

In theorizing a corporeal and sexed subjectivity that resists long-standing but false dichotomies between mind and body, Elizabeth Grosz offers the Möbius strip as a model for conceptualizing an alternative relationship between the two, a relationship of infinite interconnection, of the constant twisting and inversion of one into the other without clear beginning or end (1994). With their various examples, the Sisters in Shape women bring the Möbius strip metaphor to life through the combination of collectively determined and embodied experiences, extending its context from the mind/body relationship to one of discourse *and* embodiment; here, then, Grosz's metaphor is particularly apt in highlighting the deeply interpenetrating and mutually constitutive bases of their collective identity formation. Simultaneously drawing on their discursive as well as affective experiences in the process of articulating their group identity also allows the Sisters in Shape women to lay the groundwork for an alternative identity politics, one that develops from the coming together of what Kruks calls the "discursive spaces in which it has become possible for narratives of women's oppression and demands for recognition to emerge" (2001: 132) and the affective impetus to action. In the next chapter, I explore the multiple identity positions that this combination of discourse and embodiment makes possible.

3 / Performance

*Negotiating Multiple
Black Womanhoods*

Perhaps one of the most notable features of the Sisters in Shape women's collective identity production is its foundation in an ongoing articulation of multiple black womanhoods. At times embracing traditional black gender roles while at other times rejecting or revising them, the Sisters in Shape women continually move between and among different understandings of what it means to be a black woman. In so doing, they imagine and perform a uniquely Sisters in Shape version of black womanhood, a testament to the postmodern conceptualization of identity as discursive performance, the importance of race as an enduring and multivalent category crucial to their own identity productions, and their insistence on black women's visibility. Seemingly contradictory in their theoretical orientations, the Sisters in Shape identity performances highlight the fact that postmodern deconstructions of identity cannot account for why *black woman* is such a critical marker for the Sisters in Shape women even as they call that marker into question through their enactments of multiple identity positions with and against their essentialized, externally produced "other" representations.

These multiple instantiations of the Sisters in Shape women's identities—together with the dominant histories and ideologies that they index—foreground the political import of performative theories of subjectivity for feminist identity politics. Within feminist theories of identity, Judith Butler's work on gender performativity has been the most influential: more than any other sources (and despite the fact that she further developed these theories in later works), her books *Gender Trouble* (1990) and *Bodies that Matter* (1993) have jointly established the theoretical ground on which many others have further theorized and contested performative conceptualizations of gender, sex, and, to some degree, race. Among the most pressing questions in the debates that have arisen around these two works is that of the role of agency in discursive theories of subjectivity (a question inspired by Derrida's and Foucault's theories as well). The intentionally challenging nature of Butler's formulations leaves the question open to a range of interpretations.[1] In *Gender Trouble*, for instance, she writes that "construction is not opposed to agency; it is the necessary scene of agency" (147), and "there is no possibility for agency or reality outside of the discursive practices that give those terms the intelligibility that they have" (148). Claims such as these, which seem to locate agency in discourse rather than in individual actors, have been generative for much feminist theory even as they have inspired extensive critique; their openness to contested meanings continues to influence the already charged nature of feminist identity politics within a context of postmodernism.

In her desire to pin down individual agency in Butler's early theories of gender performativity, Sonia Kruks recuperates the significance of bodily practice by reading *Gender Trouble* through Simone de Beauvoir's embodied subjectivity, a subjectivity elaborated through the process of "becoming" a woman, a process that we might now see as similarly concerned with the emergence of subjectivity in fields of discourse and disciplinary power (2001: 70–75). Reconciling Beauvoir's theory of gender becoming with Butler's theory of performative gender, Kruks draws out Butler's implicit presumption of a subject in her argument that gender is performed under duress. If subjectivity existed only in discourse, Kruks reasons, "duress" would be irrelevant, since discourses are not vulnerable to such emotions and tensions (73). In addition, Butler's emphasis on the possibility of subversion, resistance, and slippage within discursive repetitions of gender implies "a subject that enjoys a margin of freedom within the constraints of gender production" (Kruks 2001: 74). Read together, then, Beauvoir's embodied subjectivity and Butler's performative gender offer a feminist theory of "the complex interplay of constraint *and* freedom through which gendered body-subjects both are constituted *and* constitute themselves" (Kruks 2001: 75), a theory with particular salience for the Sisters in Shape women and their distinctly embodied performances of multiple black womanhoods, performances that exploit the possibilities for freedom by resisting dominant interpellations in both discourse and bodily practice.

Before delving into those performances, however, I turn to Butler's slightly later work, particularly "Melancholy Gender/Refused Identification" ([1995] 1997), in which she continues to develop her theories of gender performance. In "Melancholy Gender/Refused Identification," Butler draws on Freud's ideas about mourning and melancholia to suggest that normative gender is achieved through a disavowal of the lost love object and the foreclosure of same-sex desire in a heterosexist society. The unresolved grief that ensues from such a foreclosure leads to a melancholic identification with (and incorporation of) the same-sex love object, the abject other. As such, Butler contends that "what is most apparently performed as gender is the sign and symptom of a pervasive disavowal" (147). In paying attention to the psychic dimensions of identity formation within the performance of gender, Butler also demonstrates that at least part of the process of subjectification occurs within the individual, though by this she certainly does not mean to suggest a coherent and stable identity position. In fact, Butler underscores the political and ethical dangers of elaborating such a position, claiming that whatever "cannot be avowed as a constitutive identification for any given subject position runs the risk not only of becoming externalized in a degraded form, but repeatedly repudiated and subject to a policy of disavowal" (149). In other words, because that which cannot be incorporated into an identity position is mapped onto the material bodies of others who come to represent the psychic exclusion, its ongoing repudiation necessarily entails the disavowal of real people. While Butler's theory of melancholy gender refers specifically to the disavowal of same-sex love and desire, it seems reasonable to extend the concept to melancholy race through the disavowal of an abject other, particularly within a racist society.

The idea that subjectivity occurs in and through identification with a repudiated other has motivated substantial theoretical insight regarding the nature of performance, embodiment, and subjectivity. One such example is Helene Moglen's innovative theorization of transageing as a concept for understanding multiple selves through the psychoanalytic concept of dissociation and her own notion of shifting "self-states of past and present" (2008: 297). Inspired by Butler's later psychoanalytic accounts of performance, subjectivity, and disavowal, Moglen investigates the political promise of identifications forged through the "interrelated consciousnesses of many selves" and argues that narratives of the self generated in such a context have the capacity to "explode the flattened, stereotypical projections of others" (308–309). Though Moglen's focus is on the individual and her multiple selves, it offers a cogent framework for considering the collective multiple selves performed by the Sisters in Shape women and the political interventions they make through such multiplicities.

I begin this chapter with this somewhat lengthy theoretical orientation in order to ground the Sisters in Shape women's multiple black womanhoods within feminist theories of performativity, discourse, and subjectification and to contextualize the specific ways that their embodied identity performances are necessarily political. Against this backdrop, I look at three specific themes—black women and black bodies; black women cooking (for themselves and others); and black women in, out of, and between groups—to explore the ways that the Sisters in Shape women move between and among different understandings of what it means to be black women, simultaneously the other of dominant U.S. culture and the ones who disavow and desire that other. These performances of an interlocking raced and gendered identity demonstrate the keen shifting that occurs as Sisters in Shape members continually constitute, if only momentarily, different notions of being a black woman—at times claiming black womanhood, at other times portraying and/or parodying black womanhood, and then at times occupying a distinctly Sisters in Shape black womanhood.

Of particular significance is the meaning that emerges between tradition and innovation in these women's performances—both discursive and practical—of black womanhood, as well as the importance that such ongoing citation and revision has for grassroots community health activism and body modification. In this context, I use the Sisters in Shape women's own discourse in my characterizations of "traditional" and "innovative" ways of embodying black womanhood, "tradition" being marked by the women's own references to "black women's practices" (both as they see themselves aligned with such practices and as they imitate other black women who participate in them) and "innovation" being their explicit recognition of how they, as Sisters in Shape members, diverge from such practices while retaining a black women's identity. I also try to situate their discourses within a broader social context so as to highlight the specific relationships that emerge when the Sisters in Shape women move between tradition and innovation in their performances to enact the activisms at the heart of the project.

Black Women and Black Bodies

The examples in this section emphasize the distinctions that the Sisters in Shape women create between themselves and "other" black women as they shift between traditional and innovative understandings of black womanhood. In this first example, which occurred during a group interview involving Melanie, Cassandra, Katrina, and Allison, Allison triggers a long discussion about the shapes and sizes of black women's bodies when she tells me a seemingly straightforward narrative of how she met Melanie and later got involved with Sisters in Shape. Before I met Allison, I used to see her training with Melanie at a local gym where I was a member. My most vivid (and favorite) memory of her is of the pained and contorted expressions on her face as Melanie subjected her to the dreaded "Butt Blaster," but equally memorable is the soft, low giggle that almost always followed the completion of her set as she and Melanie made any number of "Butt Blaster" jokes.

An executive assistant in her late 20s, Allison was about to be married when I first met her. Now, almost ten years later, she has two children, still works as a high-level executive assistant, and sometimes also works as a personal trainer for Sisters in Shape. Her memory of first meeting Melanie is deeply rooted in her (imagined) body and the ways that her literal gazing on Melanie's body in the gym inspired their meeting. At the time, one of the places where Melanie was teaching aerobics was Bally's Total Fitness in Center City, Philadelphia, a four-story gym in an old, converted building redesigned with an open core, an interior space that might have been an atrium had it been in a bank or an office building. At Bally's, this open core allowed for an extensive field of vision from almost any location in the gym as each of the three upper floors was basically constructed as a square with each side like a wide balcony, with glass half-walls, overlooking the core and the other sides of the square (the basement floor held the locker rooms). Thus, for instance, someone standing on the top floor could watch someone running on a treadmill on the second floor, as long as they were not directly above and below each other.

As a member of Bally's, Allison had been doing different types of cardiovascular exercise on her own but also wanted to begin taking some of the step aerobics classes. Not sure about the classes or the instructors, she decided to go up to the third floor, which offered an excellent view into the aerobics studio, to "check out the teacher." When she saw Melanie, she knew it would be a good class for her to take: "She walks up and I'm like, 'Oh, I could look like her,' so I started taking her class 'cause a lot of times aerobic teachers are real tiny, and, especially black women, we're thick, and lookin' at those tiny women, we're like, 'Uh, I'm not gonna look like that, you know, what's the point.'"

Here, Allison opens this narrative by explicitly positioning herself as a black woman among an imagined community of black women with similar bodies: "especially black women, we're thick." This portrayal of black women and her identification with that group comes toward the end of her introduction, however, and equally important is her initial description of seeing Melanie for the first time, as someone in whom she sees herself (potentially) mirrored. Beginning her narrative in the first person singular ("Oh, I could look like her"), Allison quickly slides into the first person plural ("especially black women, we're thick") and then, immediately in the next part of the sentence, to a combination of the two—"and lookin' at those tiny women, *we're* like, 'Uh, *I'm* not gonna look like that, you know, what's the point.'" In her discursive movement from *I* to *we* to *we/I*, Allison embeds herself in her performance of a collective and ideally imagined black womanhood—at once individual and plural—that exists in contradistinction to white womanhood as implied by "those tiny women" at the core of her narrative introduction, an identity that incorporates both the desire and the disavowal that Butler (and others) locate at the center of subject formation.

Later in this same conversation, however, the Sisters in Shape women position themselves against a differently imagined community of black women that Melanie invokes with her vivid description of black women who find personal validation (however spurious) in their male partners' comments about their bodies: "That's another problem with black women, their husbands and their boyfriends tell them, 'Oh, honey, I like you fine, with a big butt and the big thighs, you fine just the way you are.' They're not thinking about health. And unfortunately, these women feel validated through these men, and so they let these men control what they do and how they think." With comments that forge a relationship between black women's low self-esteem and black men's exploitation of that low self-esteem for control and domination (discussed in detail in the next chapter), Melanie's reference to "black women" obviously does not include the women present. Clearly Melanie, Katrina, Cassandra, and Allison are not *these* women, not the black women described in the third person *they* (unlike Allison's *we*). Entirely absent are any identifications with these women; there are no *I*'s or *we*'s here.

At this point, then, the group seems to move from Allison's initial description of an ideal black womanhood—an ideal fused with the reality of Sisters in Shape through the body of Melanie—to what they see as a more typical presentation of black womanhood as characterized by Melanie. And yet, interestingly, there are similar body features in the two presentations (at least to an observer who is not part of this immediate group)—Allison's "thick" black women do not seem too different from Melanie's women who may feel validated through the men who tell them, "Oh, honey, I like you fine, with a big butt and the big thighs, you fine just the way you are." Of course, "thick" is not necessarily "big butt and the big thighs," literally, but in both instances, "you fine just the way you are" is a fundamental part of the discourse. Indeed, the "you fine just the way you are" subtext in Allison's opening remarks, together with Melanie's comments about *these* black women, reframes Allison's initial performance and emphasizes the *ideal* nature of her imagined community of black women. That is, where Allison may seem at first to be aligning herself with a vast community of black women, she is, in fact, identifying with a more restrictive group of black women who are "thick" and who can appreciate and feel confident in that difference from white heteronormative standards of beauty.

The sense of Sisters in Shape as a different type of black womanhood is further articulated as Allison elaborates on Melanie's comments and reasserts (in slightly revised fashion) her initial characterization by using Oprah Winfrey as an example of a black woman who, according to Allison, looks good without catering to white heteronormative beauty standards. Oprah, an icon of black womanhood for Allison, becomes the focus of discussion and the mediating black body between Allison's "thick" black women and Melanie's black women with "big butt[s] and the big thighs." But Oprah does not stand alone. Allison leads into her example of Oprah as the ideal big and beautiful black woman by comparing her to Jada Pinkett-Smith, "who's real petite . . . she had a baby and she's still, she's a small woman, she's gonna be small." Moreover, Allison once again draws an imagined community of black women into the comparison between Jada Pinkett-Smith and Oprah Winfrey, suggesting that black women feel some social pressure to conform to the shape of Jada Pinkett-Smith's body, a shape largely consistent with white heteronormative body ideals: "But I don't think they realize that they don't have to look like Jada Pinkett-Smith." Rather, black women can (and should) look to other realistic black women as possible role models where body size and shape are concerned, because bodies like Oprah's suggest overall health.

Allison then goes into more specific detail, recounting some comments she heard on a local call-in radio show for black women in which the host regularly dishes about celebrities. On this particular show, a woman called in and began "mouthin' off" about how bad, how overweight, Oprah looked during one of her recent television appearances on an awards show. In somewhat uncharacteristic fashion, the show's host actually stood up for Oprah—"Hold up, I thought Oprah looked nice that night"—a point that Allison reiterates and expands to once again equate beauty with health: "And she does. She looks healthy 'cause she's probably eating better. Even if she can't exercise the way she was when she got that small, she's aware now that there's a certain way I have to eat or carry myself or do things day by day in order to be healthy . . . Even if she is twice as fat as ever, she looks healthy."

As the conversation continues, Melanie, Cassandra, and Allison all cohere around Oprah's body, extending their reading of Oprah's body to draw out Allison's earlier connection between realistic body size and overall health:

MELANIE: I saw her about two weeks ago, and I'm like, "Wow!" I know she's bigger, but she looks healthy.
ALLISON: She looks healthy. *She's the way she's supposed to be.* It's like the way, that's like the perfect size for her. [*my emphasis*]
CASSANDRA: So she's not so nutritionally starved.
MELANIE: She was all drawn before. . . . Now she full, her face is full. All those little lines, that cause that sagging, they're gone 'cause they've filled up with whatever nutrients she's getting that she wasn't getting before.

After Melanie reiterates Allison's approval of Oprah's current body shape—"bigger" but "healthy"—Allison sums it up with her contention that "she's the way she's supposed to be." Oprah, the iconic black woman, is "the way she's supposed to be," meaning bigger, fuller, "thick." Allison's own identification with this version of Oprah is made explicit as she once again slides grammatically from referring to Oprah in the third person singular to becoming Oprah in the first person singular: "Even if she can't exercise the way she was when she got that small, she's aware now that there's a certain way *I* have to eat or carry *myself*" (my emphasis).

The continual criss-crossing from tradition to innovation (and vice versa) in these performances calls attention to the complex workings of desire and disavowal, of iteration and resistance, and to the ways that meaning and identity emerge out of the actual movement *between* and *among*. That is, in this example, the Sisters in Shape women run through a series of discursive performances of race and gender, establishing first what seem to be their own expectations of what it means to be a black woman with a black body, then moving to their characterization of what they perceive to be the broader community of black women (with their attendant body issues), and then finally back to articulating their own collective position as black women with idealized relationships to their bodies. It is precisely this shifting among multiple identities that constitutes a primary mode of Sisters in Shape activism, an activism that depends on disrupting the expected raced and gendered performances of identity. Throughout the range of such performances, the Sisters in Shape women exploit the possibilities for freedom even as those possibilities are constrained by normative interpellations.[2]

In this context, then, I am suggesting that Allison's introductory performances can be read in at least two ways—first, as an identification with black women generally and, second, as a more limited identification with the type of black women involved in Sisters in Shape, in essence a disavowal of the former group. Only against the following conversation about the black women who feel validated by men claiming to like their big butts and big thighs do Allison's comments take on the second meaning. Melanie's somewhat parodic portrait of black women is, in turn, fundamental in establishing the background standard against which the Sisters in Shape women act, intervene, and ultimately resist and revise. Parody thus enables Melanie's performance, which then enables my understanding of how they, in turn, disrupt this (common) sense of being a black woman, an understanding also encoded in Allison's characterization of the black women who do not "realize they don't have to look like Jada Pinkett-Smith."

Allison's eventual move to Oprah is the key to this activist performance, the essential moment of revision that clarifies the Sisters in Shape way of being a black woman with a black body because it so clearly defines the black woman, the *we*, of her introduction as a category specific to themselves. Yet this meaning emerges only by reading Allison's introduction together with the ensuing conversations about *these* (other) black women and, later, about Oprah. Intertextually, then, the discourse on Oprah is the elaboration of Allison's introduction, the performance that opens up spaces to critique *these* black women who do not seem to get it, who continue to feel validated by the men who like their big butts and their big thighs or, alternatively, the women who do not realize they do not have to look like Jada Pinkett-Smith. Through Oprah as the representation and the embodiment of the empowered, successful, beautiful black woman who does not necessarily fit white standards of beauty, Allison, Melanie, Cassandra, and Katrina construct a particular type of black womanhood and claim it for themselves as Sisters in Shape women. More important than their self/group definition through Oprah, however, is what such a performance allows in terms of critique. For these Sisters in Shape women, one essential aspect of their collective activism exists in the ways that they resist being interpellated into the dominant category of *black women* and rupture these more common, everyday, perhaps stereotypical notions of black womanhood that damage black women's self-identity and bodily health.

Black Women Cooking (for Themselves and Others)

In this section, a much more subtle and nuanced play between tradition and innovation emerges as the same four Sisters in Shape women move through a series of performances that enact some of their various practices, attitudes, and beliefs about what it means to be a black woman cooking, for herself and others. In general, as many anthropologists and cultural studies scholars have demonstrated, cooking, eating, and sharing food all contribute to the production of both individual and group identities, the communication of values and emotions, and the negotiation of different cultural and personal beliefs across groups.[3] For the Sisters in Shape women in particular, the practice of cooking and sharing food carries with it a range of cultural meanings about not only gender but also sexuality, domesticity, history, tradition, and the construction of family and group identity.

This first example opens with two distinctly different, even opposed, perspectives on black women cooking. First, Allison introduces the topic of food shopping and preparation by referring specifically to the new context of her recently established married life. No longer cooking just for herself, she describes the occasional "flak" she gets from her husband for not preparing foods, such as fried chicken and pasta, that she herself tries not to eat. Though she rarely fried food even before she got involved with Sisters in Shape—"I wasn't good at puttin' stuff in hot grease, and it was kinda messy"—she now finds herself preparing meals for her husband that she does not eat and prefers not to cook, implying that she also cooks another, healthier meal for herself. In talking about their joint grocery shopping trips, however, Allison represents her husband as being slowly influenced by her healthier eating, forgoing pasta or choosing cookies with less fat, for instance. Though married life and cohabitation require an ongoing series of negotiations around many issues, Allison seems to be doing most of the accommodating in this particular case; her self-identified role is clearly to be the daily cook and nurturer that many Sisters in Shape members mentioned as their roles as well.

In fact, so many black women understand themselves in this role—both embracing it and complaining about it—that a central part of the official Sisters in Shape discourse (i.e., material that they produce and present) is directed at reminding black women that they should be caring for themselves as well as for everyone else, a message that is often reinforced with the point that if they are healthy, they will be better able to care for others. In this way, Sisters in Shape seeks to rearticulate the discourses of strength that confine black women to images and ideologies of "the strong black woman"—the stoic and enduring woman who not only cooks, cleans, and cares for family, community, and coworkers but who is also always available to meet the family's emotional, spiritual, and financial needs as well as the sexual needs of her (male) partner.[4] As Tamara Beauboeuf-Lafontant demonstrates in *Behind the Mask of the Strong Black Woman* (2009), black women often feel—or are made to feel—selfish if they attempt to express their emotional, physical, spiritual, familial, and/or financial needs. As a result, the women Beauboeuf-Lafontant interviewed often ignored, neglected, or abused their bodies and their psyches in their attempts to maintain the cultural mandate to be a strong black superwoman, a vexed and ambivalent representation that grants many women access to historical traditions of survival and resistance even as it authorizes continuing exploitation and oppression. In addition, many of the women in Beauboeuf-Lafontant's study suggest that performing the identity of the strong black woman renders them socially legible in a culture that would otherwise see them only as "angry," if at all. Not surprisingly, bodily and psychological neglect and abuse take their toll, and Beauboeuf-Lafontant argues persuasively that obesity and depression are two of the most common consequences of black women's attempts to live up to a damaging, unrealistic, and racist controlling image. Thus, by reminding women that they cannot care for others if they do not first care for themselves, Sisters in Shape acknowledges the prevailing discourses of strength that exist within black communities and families while also allowing women to prioritize their own health and overall well-being.

In a clear example of the Sisters in Shape rearticulation of these discourses of strength, Cassandra responds to Allison's self-presentation with her own, very different domestic scene, one in which she cooks a single meal for the entire family and insists, hypothetically, on her husband frying his own chicken if that is what he wants: "'You want some fried chicken? There's the pan, there's the chicken, fry it.' But that's how I am in my house." Before she makes this point, however, it sounds like Cassandra may be commiserating with Allison, her rejoinder to Allison beginning with the ambiguously phrased "Be unfortunate, 'cause my husband's in the same arena." Allison's background sounds of agreement further suggest that she, too, interprets Cassandra's comments as supporting her own, but it becomes more obvious as Cassandra continues that she means her husband is in the same arena that she is in. Her response then quickly becomes an alternative performance of a black woman cooking, still for herself and for someone else, but only *one* meal.

Consistent with Allison's rhetorical style as demonstrated in the previous section, she replies to Cassandra's personal example by reiterating her first point but at a slight remove from herself personally. Instead, she describes one of her clients who cooks for herself and for "the troops," the woman's nickname for her family. Sometimes it is just a little something for herself on the side, but more often than not, "she would just cook separately for 'em." Though Cassandra seems to affirm this woman's cooking practices (and implicitly Allison's) with her "okays" and "rights" interspersed throughout Allison's depiction, she eventually reasserts her strong position of not compromising in her own family and credits her long-standing commitment to cooking healthy food as the primary reason her teenage daughter Samantha has no complaints about what they have to eat. The tension at play between Allison's descriptions of black women cooking and Cassandra's portrayal of herself as a black woman cooking highlights the traditional role of primary domestic provider that many black women occupy (as do women of virtually all races and ethnicities). Significantly, the conflicting positions accord in their basic assumption of what the black woman's role is within the family; the tension exists in how one must, or can, go about fulfilling that role and the extent to which tradition may be challenged.

After Allison digresses briefly to discuss her concerns about parents teaching their children proper eating habits, I direct the conversation back to the woman who cooks for her "troops" as well as for herself. I want to know more about what the Sisters in Shape women think about her doing double duty in this way. Before I even complete my somewhat long-winded question, Cassandra cuts in with an explanation of sorts—"To keep everybody happy"—a position that Katrina quickly supports with her own claim, "It's what you gotta do." Here, then, both Cassandra and Katrina reinforce the traditional role of black women as primary domestic providers, a role that is not only assumed but also presumably inevitable if "everybody" is to remain happy, just one part of the black superwoman "job description." As a cultural outsider and a self-identified feminist, I continue to resist and suggest that it's not, in fact, "what you gotta do." In fact, to my mind, the belief that "it's what you gotta do" is a perfect example of a gender performance remaining so invisible as to maintain hegemonic structures, and I want this group of Sisters in Shape women to render the social transcript visible so they can change it. I thus press on, echoing Cassandra's perspective and suggesting that the woman not cook two meals but rather one healthy one for everyone; at this point, Cassandra and Melanie, who lives alone, offer a discursive riff on the theme with their mutual enactment of empowered, take-no-shit black women.

MELANIE: If I had a family, I would do that.
CASSANDRA: That's what I do.
MELANIE: I would be like, "Yo, I'm the boss and I'm cookin' and this is what you're eating." [*laughs*]
CASSANDRA: That's my house. Big as Jimmy is, I'm in control of that damn house.
MELANIE: "If you want something different, if you want something different, cook your own damn meal."
CASSANDRA: Exactly!
MELANIE: What's the big deal?

Melanie's and Cassandra's dual performance of what it means to be a black woman cooking recalls the energy and enthusiasm of the previous section where Allison, Katrina, Melanie, and Cassandra were constructing their own sense of being strong black women through comments about Oprah's body. In this instance, however, the Sisters in

Shape women do not reject outright what they see as the black woman's traditional role—to cook and to provide—as they did with their portrayal of the typical black women who either find validation in their men's approval of their big butts and big thighs or judge themselves by a "tiny" white heteronormative body standard. In both cases, the Sisters in Shape women interrupt the traditional sense of black womanhood and posit their own particular way of performing and embodying that identity position; here, however, the traditional category remains relatively unquestioned—that is, they do not challenge the gender expectation that women should be the primary domestic providers. What they reinvent is the way that that role is performed. In fact, maintaining their roles as caretakers remains so important that even after Melanie's and Cassandra's empowered, take-no-shit performance, the conversation takes a solidly domestic turn back toward the traditional as Katrina praises Cassandra's husband, Jimmy, after Cassandra confesses that she has never had to negotiate issues related to cooking and eating because "he just went along." Though he was not necessarily concerned with healthy eating habits when they were first married, neither was he tied to certain foods, unwilling to give them up.

KATRINA: He is such a sweetheart.
KIM: Also, probably because he didn't want to cook.
CASSANDRA: Exactly. . . . And he knew I wasn't makin' no two meals.
MELANIE: He is a good man.
CASSANDRA: He is. He is. We been together for twenty-three years.
MELANIE: She got the last good one. [*Everyone laughs.*] Ain't no more out there, girl got him.

Katrina's compliment at this moment suggests that Jimmy is a "sweetheart" precisely *because* he understands and supports Cassandra's lifestyle choices and cooking practices. But more important, perhaps, is the fact that Katrina's assertion at this moment in the conversation also opens up a full round of praise for Jimmy, which effectively reins in and tames Melanie's and Cassandra's previous take-no-shit performances. Melanie completes the cycle when she claims that Cassandra got "the last good one." This fascinating turn seems almost to police their previous conversation, unintentionally calling attention to its transgressive nature and ultimately serving as a warning or a reminder that even the strongest women must respect the boundaries of their traditional roles given the shortage of good male partners like Jimmy.

With this in mind, Cassandra returns to Allison's client who cooks for the "troops," a clear example of a woman performing her domestic duties. Cassandra, always generous in her interpretations and assessments of other people's stories, suggests that one positive way of understanding this woman's cooking two separate meals is to see it as a measure of how much energy she has now that she has started exercising and participating in Sisters in Shape. Moreover, Melanie's comments that follow offer crucial insight into the process by which tradition is acknowledged and required as part of their activist performance and commentary.

MELANIE: But you know what? It ain't that hard. She could just fry chicken for them and throw hers in the oven.
ALLISON: That's what she does.
MELANIE: She could put theirs in one pot with butter and salt and hers in another.
ALLISON: She does that.

Through these suggestions for accommodating two different eating styles at all meals, Melanie challenges her own previous performance. The pride that characterized Melanie's previous dialogue with Cassandra—her unwillingness to kowtow to others' demands that she prepare different meals for them—is referenced more obliquely here in the black woman's ability to do double duty ("It ain't that hard"), a sign of being able to do it all, being the ideal domestic partner and food provider, still being the black superwoman.

Reading and rereading the transcript of this conversation, it strikes me that the women might well have moved on to another topic at this point, but I continue to push things further; I am still not done with this woman who regularly cooks two meals. My refusal to consent to her (or any woman) doing double duty cuts through the discussion and forces the Sisters in Shape women to disrupt, once more, the immediate performance of the superbly capable family provider. My opposition is as much a feminist one as one based on Sisters in Shape's own discourses of black women's (and black families') health; I ask, yet again, why this woman should cook two separate meals when the changes she is making will likely contribute to the improved health of her own family, her troops. In addition to Melanie's and Cassandra's strong exclamations of agreement embedded throughout my own commentary, they also offer examples of an intermediate position for this woman (and themselves), not the entirely dominant have-it-my-way provider first enacted by Melanie and Cassandra, or the entirely accommodating woman who cooks two separate meals.[5] Thus, Melanie suggests that the woman may begin by communicating more thoroughly that the dietary changes she is making have more to do with preventing heart disease and possibly cancer, lowering blood pressure and cholesterol levels, and decreasing the risk of developing adult-onset diabetes, for instance, than simply with her desire to lose weight and look better. In this way, the whole family may embrace her dietary changes as important factors in their overall health status. This sort of improved health for black women *and* black families is, after all, one of Sisters in Shape's explicit goals, and Melanie continues to suggest little changes, such as switching from whole milk to skim milk or from pork bacon to turkey bacon, that this woman may make to encourage her troops to transition gradually to a healthier diet.

In this extended and lively exchange, then, Melanie moves first from an explicitly empowered reinterpretation of the traditional black woman's role as primary domestic provider ("Yo, I'm the boss and I'm cookin' and this is what you're eatin'") to a much more accommodating, unquestioning performance ("But you know what? It ain't that hard" [to cook two meals]) and finally back to a revised, though much less extreme, version of the first position. While epitomized by Melanie's performance, such discursive shifting also occurs with Cassandra, and, to a lesser degree, Katrina and Allison as well. Ultimately, the multiple selves created with this performative shifting underscore the importance of tradition to the Sisters in Shape activist discourse, as none of the women question their roles as primary cooks. Instead, they rely on that role and their potential to reinterpret the ways that they embody and practice it, thus using the traditional gender category to effect change at the broadest and most fundamental level.

Just as this group of Sisters in Shape women reinterprets the range of possibilities for performing the traditional role of primary cook and family food provider, so too do they reinvent traditional black cuisine through a shift in cooking style and method. In these cases, both the gender role and the traditional cuisine remain in place, but the means by which they are enacted and accomplished are altered in a distinctly Sisters in Shape way. In this next example, Melanie, Cassandra, Allison, and Katrina once again perform a typical Sisters in Shape health activism by drawing on tradition and innovation as counterpoints in the description of their specific cooking methods. Cassandra guides us to this part of the conversation by shifting the topic from what the woman doing double duty may do to encourage change among her "troops" to a more general concern about *how* black women are cooking: "It's hard to get the sisters to keep that fryin' pan off the stove; it's like they don't know how to do it." In response to Cassandra's critique, Allison provides some historical context while also drawing attention to the racist influences on the development of traditional black cooking in America: "Because it's, it goes so far back in our culture, of frying with the lard, we had to like make do with whatever was there." Here, Allison's comment reverberates with a claim made by Toni, another Sisters in Shape member, that African Americans generally have poor eating habits and poor health knowledge because they had to learn to cook by using whatever scraps of the pig were made available to them during slavery (discussed in detail in the next chapter).

Implicit in this brief conversational exchange is a familiar Sisters in Shape move away from a group of othered black women—the "sisters" who cannot keep the frying pan off the stove—and an almost simultaneous identification with them, at least insofar as "our culture" binds them together, the "we" who had to learn to cook with whatever bits the white slave-owners granted them. As with the earlier example in which this same group of Sisters in Shape women performed their unique identity through a complex discourse on black women's bodies, this reference to black women as a generalized group establishes the ground against which they define not only themselves but also alternative ways of preparing traditional black food. Katrina initiates a long series of examples by sharing one of the ways she prepares food differently since joining Sisters in Shape, a simple substitution that captures beautifully the tension between other black women and themselves: "They're like puttin' butter in the pan; now I have Pam."

The meaning that emerges between what *they* do and what Katrina does is further elaborated and extended in the other women's examples. Cassandra recalls a huge batch of honey-glazed chicken she made for a family picnic. Since the recipe appeared in the Sisters in Shape newsletter, the other women are familiar with it, though they have not yet tried it, and they want to know whether it is really any good. "It's delicious, it's delicious," Cassandra claims, but the real evidence comes from her extended family, who are used to fried chicken at picnics. "It went, it went just like this," she says, snapping her fingers. While she first advises the other women to prepare "healthy fare" for family functions and other potluck meals so that they themselves will always have something to eat among the other "fattenin' things," she also acknowledges the importance of introducing people to new ways of eating, to new flavors, to new foods that still fit the cultural context of a family picnic, for instance. Along these lines, she describes taking bean dip and blue corn chips to a picnic where people just stood around looking at it, put off not only by the blue chips but also by the unfamiliar bean dip: "That don't look like onion dip," she says as she imitates them puzzling over it. "It not. Try it." In the end, it turns out they are a lot like Mikey—"they like it, they like it"—though Cassandra says she also brings some yellow corn chips for those who refuse to try the blue ones. Here again, Cassandra distinguishes herself and the other Sisters in Shape women present as black women preparing healthy foods while still fulfilling their expected gender roles, the significant revision being that, unlike the other women with their frying pans, they are accomplishing slow changes in family and cultural attitudes toward healthy foods, ultimately reinterpreting the tradition while still fulfilling its social functions.

Allison refers to a similar distinction between black women and the Sisters in Shape black women, though she maps the opposition onto a generational difference as she describes the way that "older women love you puttin' butter in vegetables." She then describes her experiences with some of the older women at her church who "swore up and down that I was wrong for not puttin' butter in my vegetables." Coming together to share food after Sunday worship services, Allison and these women had long, involved conversations about the proper way to prepare the vegetables she had contributed; she prefers to steam them with herbs and perhaps a dash of oil, but the older women insisted that butter was the only way to flavor them. Short-circuiting the conversation, which could have gone on indefinitely ("They like to tell you what to do with how you cook; that's just how older women are, especially black women"), Allison finally said, "Well, did you taste these? Did you taste 'em yet?" Now, she says, when Sunday comes around they all ask, "Did you make vegetables?"

While Cassandra, Allison, Katrina, and Melanie clearly articulate the ways that they differ *in practice* from their more traditional counterparts—the sisters who cannot keep their frying pans off the stove, the ones who cook greens with pork and butter and salt—they also carefully emphasize the ways that they still fulfill their roles as black women cooking, especially for others. Thus, Cassandra cooks up healthy fare—honey-glazed chicken or bean dip with blue corn chips—for family gatherings, and Allison steams vegetables with herbs but without butter and salt for the potluck meals she attends after worship service. By situating their revised understandings of black women as primary family providers in traditional contexts such as family picnics and after-church gatherings, Cassandra and Allison stress the fundamental importance of tradition while intervening in ways that function as direct health activism. Ironically, perhaps, it is tradition that enables successful reinvention and innovation.

The movement back and forth between tradition and innovation (including that prompted by my own questions and comments) demonstrates how the specific subjectivities produced and performed in these examples—the alternating willingness and refusal to enact the scripted racialized gender roles—allow for moments of activism in the form of critical discourse, cooking practices, and the overall ways that the Sisters in Shape women "do" black womanhood differently. The tensions between Melanie's more innovative first performance and her more traditional second performance or in Cassandra's preparing healthy fare for family gatherings highlight the ways that the Sisters in Shape women rely on traditional racialized gender roles for black women in order to advance their own positions as appropriate, able, healthy, empowered, strong women while also maintaining fundamental connections to their identity communities. This activist critique is much more subtle than the example of their discourse on black women's bodies, but the ways that it simultaneously retains and revises the black woman's role as primary domestic provider may be crucial to the Sisters in Shape's widespread grassroots appeal and overall success.

Black Women in, out of, and between Groups

The examples in this last section stress the key issues—how to belong and to which communities—at stake in these varied performances of black womanhood. The tension and play between tradition and innovation and the ongoing movement back and forth between different identities so evident in the previous two sections make clear the ways that innovation absolutely depends on tradition for the success of Sisters in Shape activisms. The examples in this section thus highlight the political nature of performative identity articulated in the interplay of tradition and innovation as well as in the slippages between selves and others.

As suggested by the heading "Black Women in, out of, and between Groups," the conversations and personal narratives in this section focus on how the Sisters in Shape women create belongings and identities through their articulations of different black womanhoods. While *black womanhood* is constituted repeatedly, flexibly, differently, and momentarily in each performative iteration, its importance as an enduring identity category for the Sisters in Shape women persists, even if only abstractly imagined until specifically invoked. These examples highlight the Sisters in Shape women's concerns about belonging, about group identity (variously configured), and about negotiating the range of groups and identity affiliations of which they are (or imagine themselves to be) a part.

In the first example, I pursue this topic fairly directly, asking Joi, Nicole, and Charlie how their involvement with Sisters in Shape has influenced their relationships, both positively and negatively. In her late 40s, Joi is a fiercely intelligent transplant from Washington, D.C. She came to Sisters in Shape shortly after she arrived in Philadelphia, and the group seems to have quickly become her primary social community. At one point she even compared her feelings about other Sisters in Shape members to the feelings that soldiers develop for their comrades in wartime, a testament to her deep commitment and her perception of the challenges and hostility these women often encounter in their efforts to make major changes to their lifestyles. Of course, many soldiers would likely resist what they perceive to be the exaggerations underlying the terms of Joi's comparison; nonetheless, her analogy underscores the lack of a cultural framework for rendering intelligible both the difficulty of her lifestyle changes and the relationships that emerge out of a collective undertaking of them. Because of the intensity of her feelings about Sisters in Shape, Joi also brings a strong work ethic to the group, not just in terms of exercising but also in terms of organization-building. A core member, she has been involved with Sisters in Shape for almost ten years, and during that time she has helped organize, produce, and simply make possible the annual health and fitness symposia as well as other events such as magazine appearances, talks, and exercise demonstrations. And with the recent opening of the Sisters in Shape gym, she also spends some time working there.

Another core member and one of the first Sisters in Shape women I met, Charlie is a gentle soul, somewhat reserved at first, funny, and deeply committed to the group. More than anyone else, she now looks and seems like a different person from the one I met almost ten years ago. Charlie has lost more than one hundred pounds and dropped at least ten dress sizes, and her strength—physical, emotional, and spiritual—is apparent as she carries herself with quiet confidence. She clearly loves participating in the various aspects of Sisters in Shape: she was one of the women who first walked West River Drive with Sisters in Shape, she rarely misses any of the Saturday classes, and she is always willing to mentor new members. Without question, Charlie is a critical part of the organizational identity, and she works in whatever capacity she is needed, a reflection of her easygoing spirit. Like Joi, she has also started working at the Sisters in Shape gym, and Sisters in Shape is clearly a large part of her personal and social life. As Sisters in Shape continues to grow, and more and more women get involved, Charlie always truly symbolizes the group for me.

Nicole, in her early 30s, is much newer to Sisters in Shape than either Joi or Charlie, but she too is a core member. Nicole and her cousin Yvonne found Sisters in Shape through a seminar on black women's health held at a local hospital; inspired by Melanie and several Sisters in Shape members who came to share their stories, Nicole joined the group right away. Yvonne had just purchased a new house and was try-ing to determine whether she could afford to join Sisters in Shape, 12th Street Gym, and possibly even personal training sessions with Melanie; she initially decided that it was a bit too much to handle, but after seeing the changes Nicole had made after five or six months, she also joined. When I first interviewed Nicole, she, Yvonne, and one of their aunts were all members of Sisters in Shape and were all working out together.

In response to my question about whether their involvement with Sisters in Shape has influenced their relationships with other people, either positively or negatively, Joi begins by immediately reframing the binary choice that I present in my question and instead claims, "It's just different." This sense that "it's just different" surfaces repeatedly in her initial comments, eventually becoming amplified as a difference in how people perceive her: "So it's just different, you know, and I, I see people look at me differently." A bit later, she elaborates on who, specifically, looks at her differently—women her own age who are not in shape. Try-ing to articulate more explicitly what she means in referring to this dif-ference, she characterizes herself as being like a mirror, a comparison that begins to get at the elusive meaning: "Because they have chosen, because I have chosen a different way, so it becomes like a mirror to everyone about, um, the path that you've chosen." As mirror, Joi reflects not the other woman's own image but rather the image she has chosen not to pursue, a constant reminder of each woman's "path." With this, Joi captures beautifully the dual nature of this gazing and the ways that it firmly connects her to this other, imagined (but very real) group of women who have chosen a lifestyle that contrasts sharply to the one she has chosen. In her almost relentless attention to how her participation in Sisters in Shape (with its attendant lifestyle changes) fosters difference, Joi also establishes the boundaries between herself and what would be her peer group, "women who are my age." And while she certainly wants to register this distinction, she also seems to desire at least some affili-ation with these other women, and thus she uses the metaphor of the mirror in which they exist jointly yet separately in their mutual gaze. It is through precisely this desire for and disavowal of the other that Joi performs her identity.

In extending Joi's point to her own experiences, Nicole articulates these distinctions even more explicitly when she admits to having lost some friends who simply could not understand her desire to "put yourself through that": "That is so true, I've been through that. A couple of my friends, 'Well, why put yourself through that? You could do this at home' [*imitating them*] . . . So I had lost, um, some friends because, you know, most of my time is spent here now, but, you know, you make up for it with the people that you meet here." Joi's peer group becomes a much more intimate group in Nicole's example, but in both cases the Sisters in Shape praxis does the dual work of separating them from one group and integrating them into another. Moreover, here and throughout all the examples in this section, the separation is from a broader, more common group of black women—those who are out of shape; those who keep junk food in their desk drawers (according to Joi, who claims to work with such women); those who make all sorts of excuses about money, family, husbands; those who simply wonder why someone would undertake such seemingly difficult lifestyle changes. In the Sisters in Shape discourses, these other black women continue to contribute to the oft-cited poor health statistics for black women—such as high rates of heart disease, hypertension, adult-onset diabetes, and obesity. In articulating their differences from these women, Joi and Nicole exemplify Butler's theory of identity performance as the sign of a disavowal while also reiterating the ways that these other black women are always the abject others in the dominant imaginary and become and remain so in the Sisters in Shape imaginary.

Responding to my direct invitation to add her thoughts, Charlie continues this discourse and explores the boundaries of individual and group identity as influenced by participation in Sisters in Shape. In performing a lengthy dialogue between herself and (her imitation of) other women "our age and older," Charlie further articulates the particular Sisters in Shape black womanhood against black women much like herself.

CHARLIE: I've noticed, like a lot of women that are our age and older, they say,
CHARLIE (AS OTHER): "Oh, you look good, you know, are you still workin' out? Well, how did you do it? What did you do?"
CHARLIE: "Change the way I eat. Just change some of the things that I eat and I started working out."

CHARLIE (AS OTHER): [*exaggerated heavy sigh*] "Yeah, I know I need to go work out but it's just too hard."

CHARLIE: "No, no it's not." All you have to do is decide that this is what you wanna do, this is what you wanna do for you . . . and the first thing, you have to love yourself. If you love yourself that much, then you wanna take care of yourself and you need to take care of yourself. And takin' care of yourself means, okay, I know I need to get some exercise, and I know if I sit home I'm not gonna exercise. I don't care if I got a treadmill at home, EFX, and everything else, all you gonna do is sit home and fill clothes on top of 'em. "Uh, I don't wanna wear that today," you throw something on top of it [*two-second pause*].

CHARLIE (AS OTHER): "Well, I really don't have the money."

CHARLIE: "Well, it's really not a lot of money." Most people have insurance, and you do it through your insurance, so it's not really a lot of money. It's just excuses, and most of us have excuses why we can't.

CHARLIE (AS OTHER): "Well, I got to go home 'cause I got a family."

CHARLIE: "I have two kids. Even though they're older, I still have a family."

CHARLIE (AS OTHER): "Well, you don't have a husband."

CHARLIE: "No, I got a pain-in-the-butt man too" [*referring to her longtime partner*].

Here, Charlie notes the fine line that divides black women generally from this particular group of Sisters in Shape black women. Just as Joi refused to separate herself entirely from a larger, more common group of black women (women her age but out of shape), Charlie likewise draws out the similarities between herself and other women her age even as she distinguishes herself from them by referring to her participation in Sisters in Shape—they are all prone to excuses, they all find exercising a challenge and could easily talk themselves out of it, they all have family responsibilities. Her lengthy dialogue captures her and Joi's subtle desire to affiliate with a group from which they also want to remain separate. Along these lines, Charlie's parodic description of these other black women's excuses eventually fuses with her own when she moves from the second person to the first person and says, "Okay, I know I need to get some exercise and I know if I sit home I'm not gonna exercise. I don't care if I got a treadmill at home, EFX, and everything else." She is, simultaneously, one and the other.

The simultaneous avowal and disavowal of this other group of black women is of fundamental importance for the Sisters in Shape members, a point that Joi makes when she describes her way of turning down (junk) food offered to her: "I don't want to make that separation, you know, where people start to feel that I feel better or, you know . . . [*trails off*]"—and here Charlie takes advantage of Joi's slight pause to complete the thought by adding "you're better than them." "Exactly," Joi says as she picks up where she left off, "so I just, you know, I don't say anything." Here, then, is the crux of these related excerpts: separation is both desired and resisted. Unlike some gender activists who seek to be entirely subversive, who want to confuse gender so as to abolish gender categories altogether (and for whom gender preempts race and is most frequently theorized from an unmarked racial position), these Sisters in Shape women seek, instead, to revise the identity category—black women—to which they belong and to which they want to continue belonging. In many ways, the Sisters in Shape movement is about black body pride, about being a strong healthy black woman with high self-esteem. Thus, for the Sisters in Shape women, the category remains unchallenged; the challenge, rather, is how to embody the position, how to live and claim the differences without making the separation.

In similar fashion, Katrina also moves back and forth between different black womanhoods, ultimately establishing an innovative position to demonstrate how activism emerges from the Sisters in Shape sense of sisterhood but also underscoring the importance of simultaneously identifying with those whose othering furthers their group production. A tall, thin woman in her mid-20s, Katrina found Sisters in Shape after seeing Melanie in an aerobics demonstration. As a former dancer, Katrina loved the demonstration and was inspired, much as Allison was, by the possibility of developing her body's musculature and perhaps one day looking like Melanie. Talking together after the demonstration, they realized they had many common interests, and Katrina claims she felt immediately drawn to Melanie, whom she describes as her "surrogate mother."

Katrina has a sweet, soft personality, and though she seemed a bit shy in formal interview contexts, she was able to open up, laugh, and joke as she began to feel more and more comfortable with me and the process of recording our conversations. One of Katrina's most endearing qualities is her impishness, the way she almost laughs at herself as she says something she knows the others will respond to, enjoying her own naughtiness as much as she enjoys gently goading them on. On one occasion, I remember her walking in a bit late to our group interview, which was already under way. The other women stopped to greet her, remarking on her new hairstyle and her fashionable and figure-flattering clothes. When asked about her shirt, a men's tank top undershirt, Katrina said, "Yeah, this is called a 'wife-beater,'" knowing that Cassandra would give her a little lecture about the term. Her eyes twinkled as she waited for Cassandra's response, a fairly long rant about the name and the vile nature of domestic abusers. In many ways, her playfulness is a marker (for herself especially) of the group's closeness, a sign of the cherished "sisterhood" she finds with Sisters in Shape.

Responding to one of my direct questions about Sisters in Shape's ability to cultivate a sense of sisterhood, an aspect of the group that many of the women mentioned as critical to their participation in it, Katrina immediately separates Sisters in Shape from other groups of black women: "I love it [the sisterhood quality]—because it's so uncommon, especially amongst African American females. It's always some type of problem; it's always jealousy, whether it's hidden or whether they're displaying it." She then begins to cite various examples of what sisterhood means in the context of her Sisters in Shape experiences: first, it seems to be a general and sincere caring for each other, a recognition of the other women's feelings and moods and a real interest in those feelings; second, it is a deep identification with each other, with the changes that they are all trying to incorporate into their lives; and third, it is a particular energy they generate when they are all together. Most important, though, it seems to be the way that all of those factors come together in a discourse and practice of self-care and health, and this aspect truly seems to separate Sisters in Shape, at least in Katrina's mind, from other black women: "And the fact that these African American women—because we are basically lazy, you know, we are, African

American women are lazy—but to have these women who care about themselves and they have the same interests. And we don't take this lightly; we take this very seriously."

Moreover, according to Katrina, the Sisters in Shape women can come together to support each other because the group gives them a certain confidence that sets them apart from other black women, a confidence that allows them to support each other without feeling threatened in their own goals and identities. She compares her experiences with Sisters in Shape to her earlier experiences dancing to further illustrate her point. The dancers will "trip you in a minute . . . they'll stab you in the back in a minute"; she remembers some of them saying things to her like, "Oh, look at your gut, why don't you suck that gut in?" With Sisters in Shape, on the other hand, "it's just like everybody's not interested in competition," preferring instead to build each other up as they work together toward common goals, sharing compliments instead of shaming each other: "We are open; we feel that we can go to each other and say, 'You lookin' good, your ass lookin' good . . . you are so gorgeous,' you know, and I have no problem with that."

In describing African American women as lazy, Katrina first aligns herself with the broader identity category ("we are basically lazy") and then immediately distances herself from that category by invoking a different collectivity: "but to have these women who care about themselves." Katrina's shift from *we* as black women to "*these* black women who care about themselves" marks the differences as well as the affiliations so crucial to the production of Sisters in Shape black womanhood as a unique identity construct. What's more, Katrina's stark contrast between dancers and Sisters in Shape members reiterates the group's separation from the broadest category of African American women— characterized here as lazy, jealous, competitive, aggressive, and lacking in confidence—even as it enables a reinterpretation of that identity on a group level. Thus, just as the Sisters in Shape women can perform their gendered roles through individual acts of food preparation or through conversations about black women's bodies, Katrina suggests that Sisters in Shape, as a group, can still be bound and defined by the descriptor *black women*, can still identify as and with black women generally, even as they strive to alter many of the traits traditionally associated with groups of black women.

For the Sisters in Shape women, intervention into and recuperation of the generally imagined category of *black woman* is crucial to their own belonging, a belonging that brings them together and keeps them together, as "sisters" in shape working toward the same sorts of lifestyle changes. At the same time, it is the essence of their activism, the point from which they depart. That is, in revising—performatively in discourse and bodily in praxis—but not dismantling the category of *black woman*, these Sisters in Shape members take activist stands on a range of issues, including black women's health, self-esteem, relationship with white heteronormative standards of beauty, and public images. Because the Sisters in Shape women are part of the larger community (in the imagination and in the reality of their everyday lives)—their activism thrives in between. The deep and fundamental level of activism that exists between a more everyday sense of black womanhood and the Sisters in Shape revision of that identity category creates the basis and the appeal of the Sisters in Shape movement and highlights their enduring commitments to traditional and innovative ways of performing their embodied identities.

As the examples in this chapter illustrate, the Sisters in Shape women perform their identities against and through an abject other who is also their intimate and uncanny twin, the black woman through whose repudiation white (female) Americans come to define themselves. It is this dominant interpellation that the Sisters in Shape women resist, the hail they refuse to answer as they choose, instead, to exercise their freedom within constraint by revising the category of the black woman. Ironically, as the Sisters in Shape women make clear, performative theories of subjectivity provide crucial insight into the importance of identity categories. For Sisters in Shape, the identity category itself proves central to their activism and political intervention precisely because it draws attention to the long-standing cultural disavowal of black women in a racist society. Without the identity category, the Sisters in Shape revisions and subversions are simply unintelligible; with the identity category, their performances—both discursive and embodied, the "being" and the "doing"—generate alternative subject positions capable in turn of generating social and political change.

4 / New Bodies of Knowledge

Hegemonic ideologies of the body are often rendered visible when "othered" bodies are drawn into dominant discourses, made to serve as points of comparison. For instance, the process by which it has become almost common knowledge that black women are more comfortable with their bodies than are white women reveals some of the white heteronormative body ideologies that maintain black women's invisibility and poor health in a racist and sexist culture. This chapter centers on the Sisters in Shape women's explicit interventions into dominant explanations of black women's higher body esteem as compared to white women's and builds on the previous two chapters to explore the ways that the Sisters in Shape women generate a unique black feminist standpoint that resists reinforcing a fixed identity.

Standpoint theory has been crucial in challenging hegemonic feminist theories and epistemologies by drawing from a greater diversity of experiences and by developing more nuanced accounts based in intersectional analyses. The widespread and diverse critiques of "second-wave" feminism as exclusive of the knowledges and experiences of women who are positioned in nonhegemonic social locations—determined by race, ethnicity, class, sexuality, ability, age, and citizenship, among other identity markers—attest to the power of standpoint theory. Along these lines,

Patricia Hill Collins (1991, 1998), bell hooks (1981, 1990), Angela Davis (1981), and Audre Lorde (1984) have delineated the importance of black women's experiences to black feminist thought. Underlying their work and the extensive work they have inspired, however, is the tendency to reinscribe a fixed group identity, an enduring category of *black women* that implies a stable self at its center. By bringing together a set of collective experiences based in both discourse and embodiment (discussed in Chapter 2) and an understanding of Sisters in Shape's particular black womanhoods as performative and multiple (discussed in Chapter 3), the women of Sisters in Shape recover the promise of standpoint theory for subject formation, political consciousness, feminist epistemology, and social and political change. Against the hegemonic assumptions that black women have greater body esteem than do white women because of different cultural standards, I read a range of Sisters in Shape discourses as a complex cultural commentary that reorients the dominant discourse of black women's higher body valuation and rearticulates alternative ways of understanding self-esteem in relation to race and the body. Throughout this chapter, I foreground the Sisters in Shape women's interventions in order to highlight the ways that their multiple and embodied selves prompt us to reconsider the complex interworkings of "women's experiences" to feminist theory and feminist activisms as well as the relationship of particular standpoints to new bodies of knowledge.

The Sisters in Shape women's experiences as simultaneously discursively constituted and embodied sources of knowledge exemplify Satya P. Mohanty's understanding of experience as crucial to a reinvigorated standpoint theory and to the generation of alternative epistemologies (1993). In suggesting a productive return to the intersection of experience, identity formation, and feminist standpoint theory for social and political change, Mohanty seeks to mediate some of the tensions between difference feminists and postmodern feminists around identity politics, particularly in terms of the debate between essentialism and radical constructivism. Given his contention that experiences can be assessed like any other form of knowledge, Mohanty finds a solution in an objective (or critically evaluated) feminist standpoint. According to Mohanty, an objective feminist standpoint develops out of an understanding of "women's experiences" as a theoretical concept grounded in and constrained by a gender-stratified society, an understanding that grants the socially constructed nature of "women's experiences" while recognizing the ways that such experiences can be evaluated in order to serve as objective forms of knowledge (as discussed in Chapter 2). Such an argument resonates with Nancy Hartsock's now-classic definition of feminist standpoint as distinct from women's standpoint more generally; feminist standpoint, according to Hartsock, undertakes a critical analysis of the dominant social practices that sustain women's oppressions in order to articulate a different social reality that might liberate all people (1985, 1998). Despite her important vision for human emancipation through feminist standpoint theory, Hartsock generally relies on an overly universalizing understanding of the "feminists" who generate her feminist standpoint. Expanding on Hartsock's universal "feminists" by focusing on black women in particular, Patricia Hill Collins describes the specific ways in which black women's experiences generate black feminist theory (1991, 1998). For Collins, a black feminist standpoint moves beyond traditional identity politics that fix groups in relation to a normative center; rather, she relies on intersectionality—with its emphasis on the co-constitutive nature of different social categories—to argue for *black women* as a complex but definable category that captures "the historical realities that created and maintain African-American women's particular history . . . while recognizing the complexity that operates within the term" (1998: 152–153).

While Mohanty, Hartsock, and Collins all make important contributions to feminist theories of identity and identity politics with their attention to particular feminist standpoints, none go far enough in addressing the multiple dimensions of the postmodern critique. Because Mohanty conceives of the debates over identity as primarily hinging on the status of experience (i.e., experience as either "real" and unifying or socially constructed and arbitrary), he never accounts for the status of the subject vis-à-vis social constructionism, focusing instead on the political import of rethinking dominant theories of experience. Similarly, while Collins's articulation of a complex category of *black women* and her description of a black feminist standpoint as informed by intersectionality are much more nuanced than earlier theorizations (including her own), they nonetheless continue to imply an identifiable and shared subjectivity at the center of the category. For many postmodern feminists, this stability undermines standpoint theory regardless of whether groups overgeneralize collective experience or are fixed in relation to a normative center.

Addressing many of these concerns while seeking to account for the radical historical and cultural contingencies implicit in multiple feminist epistemologies, Donna Haraway develops a theory of standpoint defined by "situated knowledge" and feminist objectivity. As Haraway argues, situated knowledges and reflexive positionalities are necessarily embodied and partial; as such, they are also locatable within "webs of connections called solidarity in politics and shared conversations in epistemology" (1988: 584), and an informed recognition of situatedness allows for a kind of objectivity. Haraway's theory of situated knowledges and partial vision is especially relevant for rethinking identity politics because it insists on the impossibility of *being* and *seeing* simultaneously: "One cannot 'be' either a cell or molecule—or a woman, colonized person, laborer, and so on—if one intends to see from these positions critically. 'Being' is much more problematic and contingent. Also, one cannot relocate in any possible vantage point without being accountable for that movement" (585). For Haraway, then, standpoint and identity must be mobile and shifting, not so much a fixed identity position as a self-conscious and momentary location from which to see. Through their ongoing performances of multiple and shifting black womanhoods, the Sisters in Shape women bring to life Haraway's theory of situated knowledge, thus offering one possible way of recuperating the power and political promise of feminist standpoint theory without reinforcing an enduring or consistent black womanhood. Instead, they suggest a series of group-based identity standpoints—rooted in Haraway's partial perspectives and feminist objectivity—in lieu of a singular black women's standpoint. In this chapter, I explore one such Sisters in Shape standpoint as it emerges in their discourses about body esteem, thus highlighting the importance of standpoint theory to the development of new epistemologies.

Shape, Size, and Self-Esteem: A Portrait in Black and White

Throughout the academic and popular literatures and among the Sisters in Shape women's discourses—as reflected in conversations, personal narratives, and interviews—self-esteem is assumed to be something individuals possess, albeit to varying degrees. None of the academic researchers, journalists, or Sisters in Shape women critically interrogate self-esteem as a social construct articulated with normalizing ideologies. Because the Sisters in Shape women intervene in dominant discourses of black women's bodies as specifically linked to self-esteem (all of which assume its "real" basis), I choose to work alongside and within those assumptions in this chapter; in the next chapter, however, I push against this largely unquestioned acceptance of self-esteem as a way of further engaging the questions of group identity and social and political change at the heart of *Body Language*.

The fascination with white and black women's differing levels of self-esteem in relation to their bodies is extensive. Drawing on information from numerous research studies in disciplines such as nursing, medicine, public health, social work, and psychology,[1] popular sources such as *Essence* and the *New York Times* have spread the word that black women tend to have higher body esteem than do white women even as more culturally sensitive sociological studies offer a range of nuanced insights into and perspectives on disordered eating among African American, Latina, and white women (e.g., B. Thompson 1994; Logio 2003; and Beauboeuf-Lafontant 2003, 2009). For instance, Becky W. Thompson's seminal work *A Hunger So Wide and So Deep* (1994) challenges the prevailing belief that eating disorders are largely the concern of young, white, middle-class, heterosexual women concerned with body appearance. By sharing the life stories of diverse African American, Latina, and white women—women of different social classes, sexual identities, religious backgrounds, and immigration status—Thompson reorients the dominant perception of eating disorders by highlighting the ways that "eating problems" (Thompson's more neutral nomenclature for compulsive overeating, bingeing, bulimia, anorexia, and restrictive dieting) often function as survival strategies against a range of physical and emotional abuses in these women's lives. At the same time, she is careful not to romanticize such practices as unproblematic acts of resistance, and she draws on the women's own reflections to illustrate how an initial survival strategy can easily become an unhealthy and damaging force. Through a truly diverse selection of women's stories, Thompson advances the idea that eating problems are about much more than body image, and her attention to a multiracial analysis usefully expands the standard comparison of black and white women.

Despite these types of careful, culturally sensitive studies that explore the multidimensional ways that social, cultural, and personal traumas and expectations motivate eating problems such as compulsive overeating, bingeing, and bulimia, mainstream accounts most frequently return to and reinforce the purported differences between black and white women's body esteem. Thus, although *Essence* and the *New York Times*, for example, invoke such studies in slightly different contexts and read different meanings into and out of them, the bottom line is oft-cited and persistent: regardless of size, shape, and weight, black women simply have less body dissatisfaction and higher self-esteem than do white women.

In a 2000 *New York Times* article, for instance, Natalie Angier refers to one study in which black women expressed body dissatisfaction only when their body mass index (BMI) scores approached the "obese" category, whereas white women expressed body dissatisfaction as their BMI scores neared the "overweight" category. Angier uses this study to stress the fact that different cultural factors underlie the overall national (i.e., across racial/ethnic groups, class, sex, and geographical lines), and even worldwide, increase in obesity, and she highlights the paradox that while positive self-esteem is certainly good for black women's mental health, greater body satisfaction at higher weight may not be so good for their physical health.[2]

By comparison, *Essence* magazine's discussion of its 2001 online survey of self-selected participants celebrates black women's attitudes toward their bodies and especially their redefinition of a "great body" as *not* a waif (Scruggs 2001: 94). Afi-Odelia Scruggs highlights the cultural pride implicit in this (re)definition—*not* a waif—which specifically reorients the predominant white heteronormative standard for a "great body" as represented in mainstream media, a point that she further reiterates by invoking the wisdom of her group in the form of a proverb: "We have a saying of our own: Nobody but a dog wants a bone" (2001: 94). Both of Scruggs's articles, which clearly presuppose a black group identity and audience, read like happy declarations of resistance to white heteronormative body standards, a tone echoed in Ziba Kashef's accompanying article summarizing the results of the online reader survey. Kashef opens with three anonymous quotations from the survey as a collective epigraph: "I'm pretty much at peace with the body I have";

"I am happy with my own body but want to improve it"; "I love my body!" (2001: 96). Though Kashef goes on to complicate this picture by citing women's complaints about their bodies, the three opening quotations best convey the overriding tone. The third, and briefest, article in this *Essence* feature goes on to discuss the "perfect body" in terms of health, offering general suggestions for healthy living, including advice to exercise, reduce stress, quit smoking, and refrain from drinking excessively (Shelton 2001: 98).

At the same time, *Essence* has continually addressed obesity and overeating among its readership (e.g., Weathers 2003a, 2003b; Powers 1989; Gregory 1997; Anonymous 2004; and Phillips and Gregory 1997), thus creating the social space necessary for understanding eating practices as indexes of more than self-control. By interrogating the practices as well as the discourses of overeating, *Essence* helps its readers see themselves as part of a group of women who may turn to eating as a survival strategy in the face of personal and social abuses and oppressions. Both Becky Thompson (1994) and Tamara Beauboeuf-Lafontant (2003, 2009) describe the ways that women's eating problems begin as modes of survival, comfort, and resistance but later slip into destructive practices. By raising awareness around some of the possible motivations for compulsive overeating and obesity, *Essence* may begin to shift black women's awareness of their own relationships to food even as they grapple with internalized standards for "properly" (i.e., heteronormative) gendered, raced, and sexed body shapes and sizes. Self-esteem runs through all of these discourses on the body as women negotiate feminist, sexed, cultural, individual, and hegemonic ideals and ideologies about their bodies, beliefs that deeply influence how they understand them, how they feel about them, and how they live with and within them.

The Sisters in Shape discourse is also replete with discussions of self-esteem and body (dis)satisfaction, but the conversations differ radically from those most frequently cited in academic research literature and the popular media. In the following narratives drawn from my interviews with the Sisters in Shape women about a wide range of topics, they clearly not only contest and resist the assumptions and assertions grounded in white heteronormative ideologies of the body but also completely shift the grounds of the discussion as they produce their own theories about the relationship of race, gender, body image, and self-esteem.

Controlling Factors: Black Women's Body Valuation at the Intersection of Sex and Race

Despite the interventions of culturally sensitive studies of black women and disordered eating such as those mentioned previously, the most frequently cited studies—both academic and popular—are still largely preoccupied with black and white women's differing body valuations and self-esteem. Within this context, one of the most dominant tropes centers on black men's appreciation and sexualization of larger women, an aesthetic frequently posited as a primary reason for black women's greater body esteem. Indeed, one of the first claims made in the *Essence* article on black women's bodies and black women's self-esteem announces this belief in clear and explicit terms: "Black men like butts, breasts and bigger bodies. Larger Black women get positive feedback from our men of color" (Greene, quoted in Scruggs 2001: 90). Likewise, Allan, Mayo, and Michel (1993) report that the black women in their study of body-size values among black and white women held similar beliefs: "Overweight and obese black women stated the men in their lives thought they looked just fine and preferred them 'healthy' and larger. A black woman described her partner's preference for her body size and shape: 'I have big hips, a big butt, and a small waist. The guys love it and they would never say I was fat'" (331). Comments like these give the impression of a deep and widespread set of community beauty standards, standards that are valued by both men and women and that are understood by researchers and reporters to contribute to black women's higher self-esteem in relation to their bodies, especially when their bodies do not fit idealized white heteronormative beauty standards.

At the same time, however, assumptions about the popularity of such beliefs may blind many researchers to the more subtle ways that some black women may resist the overarching nature of these claims, refusing to situate themselves wholly in these discourses. For instance, Allan, Mayo, and Michel (1993) report another woman's perspective as a second example of black women's supposed internalization of black men's preference for larger women: "Another woman said, 'You *handle* weight when you are heavy because you have this boyfriend telling you that you look good with that weight on you'" (331; my emphasis). While the researchers understand this as yet another example of a "heavy" black woman with positive body values, I want to read this woman's comments against the researchers' interpretation by suggesting that she invokes the word *handle* in this context to mean that being "heavy" is a burden, a challenge, something that requires conscious rationalization—emotional or psychological *handling*—in order to cope with it. One way of coping, or handling, her being heavy is through the approval of her boyfriend, or of men generally, but there seems to be a clear distinction in her comments between her boyfriend's and her own body valuation.

I draw out my reading of this woman's remarks against the researchers' understanding of them to question the dominant discourse of cultural homogeneity regarding the fullness of black women's bodies. While such an idea may be rooted in the everyday lived realities of many black men and women, sustained attention to it seems to obscure other issues at play in black men's supposed love of big black women. In this section, I draw from interviews with several Sisters in Shape women who comment specifically on this discourse to reinterpret the meanings embedded in black men's claims to love their women big. They critique not only black men but also the ways that researchers have presented other black women's interpretations of black men's comments. In so doing, they also produce significant theories of how sexism and misogyny operate through others' discourses about their bodies.

In one group-interview setting, Melanie specifically raises this issue by moving our group discussion in this direction, using my presence as an opportunity to critique men who fail to support their partners, a criticism she and other Sisters in Shape women eventually connect to the same men who supposedly love big women. She begins by calling my attention to the importance of the example she is about to share—"Another thing, Kim, worth mentioning"—and then tells an all-too-familiar story about one of her clients, Kathryn, a story that reiterates the social expectations that black women must perform the role of a superwoman without attending to (or indeed having) needs of their own. I have never met Kathryn, but I know from Melanie that she is married with children, works outside the home, and has struggled to find the time to participate fully in Sisters in Shape. Though she is a member of the group, she rarely attends the Saturday exercise classes or the rap sessions that follow, and she spends most of her gym time lifting weights in personal-training sessions with Melanie. After a few weeks of difficulty keeping appointments and constantly shifting her schedule, Kathryn arrived one night for a session with Melanie; she rushed into the gym, huffing and puffing, her frantic "Okay, let's work out" signaling to Melanie that her workout was just another thing on a long list of things to do, what Dworkin and Messner have termed the "third shift" because of the cultural pressure on women (especially white middle-class women) to maintain their bodies in addition to their other responsibilities (1999). Before beginning, Melanie asked her why she was so rushed, and Kathryn's simple rehearsal of her day—going straight from work to pick up the kids, rushing them home, getting them settled in with snacks and homework and activities, preparing things for dinner later, then heading back downtown to the gym—was explanation enough.

In response to Kathryn's account of her day, Melanie asked her a series of further questions that underscores Sisters in Shape's attempts to disrupt the myth of the black superwoman by authorizing the choice black women may make to pay attention to themselves and their own needs: Why did your husband not pick up the kids? Or get the meal started? Or get them settled in after school? Why does your husband not watch the kids at other times so you can have a more convenient appointment time? Kathryn did not really have any answers, at least not any Melanie thought sufficient: "You know, it was not a good reason, no, no good reason." Immediately following her assessment of Kathryn's husband's excuses, Melanie went on to link his utter lack of support to his desire to keep his wife's self-esteem low: "You know what the problem is, in a lot of these cases, is that the men, they don't want their women to go and get their acts together. They want their self-esteem to remain low so that they can remain in control. They don't want them to get smaller and look really good and fierce and think better about themselves because they don't want to increase their risk of their cheating on them." Cassandra, a core Sisters in Shape member also present during this interview, echoed Melanie's assertion, suggesting that such men "don't want other men lookin' at them [their wives]." With a hope of future empowerment for women like Kathryn, Cassandra then moves the critique in a more positive direction, claiming that with physical strength will come mental strength. She completes her claim by imagining what a woman who has garnered that strength may say: "I don't need you. I had to pick up the kids, cook the dinner, do that, get my workouts, and now I'm lookin' good. You can just go on and get out of my life 'cause you haven't done a thing."

Melanie offers this narrative of a woman whose partner provides no support for her participation in Sisters in Shape as an example of what she sees as a significant issue for many black women. By taking control of our conversation to raise this specific concern, Melanie gives weight to the story and to the theory that she and Cassandra generate from it. After providing the details of Kathryn's case, she summarizes the problem as men's desire to control the women in their lives by maintaining the women's low self-esteem. Though Kathryn's husband's attitudes toward her body are explicitly absent from this narrative, Melanie makes explicit the logic she ascribes to Kathryn's husband and to black men in general: "They don't want them to get smaller and look really good and fierce." That is, as long as Kathryn (and women like her) remain big, other men will not be as tempted by them, implying a beauty standard that values smaller women. In this comment, then, Melanie not only critiques Kathryn's husband and other black men like him but also contests the common belief that most black men and women value larger black women; she herself equates looking "really good and fierce" with being "smaller" and suggests that many black men do as well.

Perhaps most significant in this narrative, though, is the motivation that Melanie and Cassandra ascribe to black men's supposed love of big black women, specifically the desire to maintain their positions of control. Melanie's logic is direct and to the point: these men can remain in control only if the women have low self-esteem. In this way, Melanie recasts black men's supposed love and appreciation of black women's big bodies by proposing the idea that black men *use* this cultural ideal to keep heavy black women's self-esteem low, thereby making it easier for them to control these women. This alternative understanding of black men's positive valuation of black women's larger bodies also provides a context for a better understanding of the woman cited in Allan, Mayo, and Michel (1993) who "handled" her being heavy through interactions with men; indeed, Melanie's position gives meaning to the seeming disjuncture between that woman's conceptualization of being heavy as a burden or a challenge and her rationalization of it through male discourses on her body. As Melanie makes clear, those discourses feed the disjuncture and ensure that such women continue to "handle" their heaviness not with exercise and healthy living but by doing nothing.

For Melanie and Cassandra, *control* takes on many meanings when they describe the ways that black men maintain their control over black women by sustaining their low self-esteem. On the most literal level in this narrative, *control* has to do with the domestic hierarchy of the relationship itself; Kathryn's husband apparently has the power to determine who does what domestic work, and Kathryn's health and well-being suffer under this unbalanced distribution of labor. On another literal level, *control* is about the woman's body and who can view it, touch it, have sex with it. As Cassandra said, these men "don't want other men lookin' at them [their female partners]." But *control* also takes on more nuanced meanings. Cassandra's inspired claim that "with the physical strength will come mental strength" indexes a much more elusive understanding of *control*, a psychological and emotional control requiring mental strength to escape, a point she also makes as she imagines a future in which these women gain the strength—physical, mental, spiritual—to leave their partners, who simply cannot support them, with a parting shot.[3]

Through these elaborations of what *control* means and how black men maintain it in the contexts of their relationships with big black women, Melanie and Cassandra make explicit the links among body, self-esteem, and black women's oppression on individual and social levels. They are not willing to stand for black men's love of big black women as an excuse for male domination and control; nor are they willing to stand for black men's love of big black women as an excuse for remaining overweight and unhealthy. Theorizing from the ground, from their lived experiences and the shared experiences of other women they know, Melanie and Cassandra powerfully reinterpret black men's love of big black women to critique the misogyny and sexism that damage not only black women's self-esteem and mental health but also their physical health, quality of life, and overall wellness.

Of course, to critique black men's love of black women with full, large, round bodies is not to suggest that they do not, in fact, love these features in black women's bodies. That is, I am not suggesting a false or intentionally misleading love of shapely bodies or calling for a body ideal that approaches white heteronormative beauty standards. Rather, I, along with Melanie and Cassandra, am calling attention to the potentially dangerous subtexts within these discourses and positing healthy, muscular, strong, full bodies as alternatives to unhealthy, overweight bodies linked to women's low self-esteem and to men's domination. However, as Cassandra makes clear through her own story, not all black men may be interested in that alternative.

In one of our early interviews, Cassandra tells Melanie and me that she has noticed a difference in how black men respond to her on the street now that she is leaner and more muscular: "African American men look at me and turn their head [away]. I get more attention from white men." Cassandra understands these differences—black men turning their heads from her when they would have ogled her before, and white men now noticing her—as related to her leaner, more muscular body's ability to signal strength, a strength she feels black men are not interested in. "It's that strength," she says, and she goes on to describe her particular way of walking: "And you know how I walk; I do have a certain walk. I walk the way I feel." Melanie and I confirm her "certain walk," comparing her to mythical African royalty, and in response Cassandra reiterates her earlier point about black men ignoring her on the street—"[They] just don't even look at me. Man, they like, ppbbhhh"—and then moves into an imitation of them: "She gonna be expectin' too much." In the end, she herself analyzes their motives: "It's more like I'm a threat to 'em. . . . They lookin' for something different, I guess." Melanie and another core member, Allison, concur, and Melanie's comment once again exemplifies the relationship that these women perceive between women's self-esteem and men's insecurities and, thus, desire for control: "That's probably because the only kinda woman that they can get are those that have no self-esteem." Allison further characterizes these women as "walkin' with their head down in their shoulders," an image diametrically opposed to Cassandra's proud walk, head held high. Cassandra and Melanie end the conversation at the same moment, Cassandra referring to herself when she says "too much muscle" (for the men who ignore her) and Melanie summing it all up with a single word: "yeah, *control*."

Though Cassandra's and Kathryn's stories differ remarkably in their characterizations of the two women's levels of empowerment, they both generate essentially the same discourse on black men's need for control in relation to black women's bodies and black women's self-esteem.

Cassandra sees these black men who ignore her on the street as threatened by her, by her public movements, by her explicit markers of strength. She imagines them thinking that "she gonna be expectin' too much." The discourse on black men's need to control women becomes especially clear in Melanie's responses to Cassandra, in her support of her "regal" walk, her public presence, her strong body. Distinguishing Cassandra from the women with no self-esteem, the women who walk with their heads down in their shoulders, Melanie and Allison echo the concerns that emerge in Melanie's discussion of Kathryn.

And yet, equally significant are the ways that this conversation about black men's sexism and misogyny is inflected with race: "Since I've gotten leaner like this, African American men look at me and turn their head [away]. I get more attention from white men." While Cassandra's opening statement is certainly about African American men, it cannot be separated from her immediate comparison of African American men to white men. In this brief mention of white men, the sole reference to them in this entire interview (possibly all the interviews), Cassandra speaks volumes on the racial aspects of black men's sexism. In the logic of these two stories, black men seem to need control over "their" women, at least on the level of individual relationships; they do not want women who feel good about themselves, strong women who may be equal and, thus, willing to challenge such things as the domestic division of labor and the psychological and emotional domination that benefits black men. At the same time, Cassandra also implies that white men do not need this same control; after all, they are now looking at her. While white men may have different beauty standards and body ideals for women than do black men, those standards may still index issues of control in relation to women. Given their privileged social status, white men may assume they already have the type of control that Cassandra suggests black men desire; thus, according to her implicit logic, white men have no reason to be threatened by her public presence and her strength. In the end, Cassandra's discourse comparing black men and white men calls attention to a racial hierarchy in which black men are implied to be less confident than white men, less able to handle a strong black woman (which, of course, accords with the general racism of our society wherein male privilege and entitlement correspond with race and class status).

In integrating the racial aspects of black men's sexism into their discussions, Cassandra and Melanie expound a complex theory of intersecting and interlocking modes of oppression that directly affect black women's bodies. At the same time, they create an opportunity for critiquing black men's misogyny—something they frequently encounter—and invite comparison to white men as a way of further expressing their strength as black women in relation to black men. After all, comparing black men to white men effectively does to black men what those same men seem to do to black women, namely to chip away at their self-esteem so as to better dominate them. Melanie's and Cassandra's theorizing of this point beautifully demonstrates the sad fact of racial oppression and the way it furthers gender oppression through black women's bodies.

Perceived Gazes: The Gym and the Social Mirror

Running throughout the Sisters in Shape discourses on self-esteem is an exploration of the tension at play between the individual concerns and the institutional conditions that frame, structure, and at times even determine the ways that race, body, and self-esteem ultimately intersect. While much of the mainstream academic research and popular reports mention both personal and cultural factors in their comparisons of black and white women's varying body valuations, the Sisters in Shape women exploit these same factors specifically as a tension in order to create a key discursive register for asserting their own theories and for generating new paradigms for black women's visibility within the context of health and fitness.

In this section, the gym is situated as a literal and symbolic space joining the personal and the institutional. Discussing the ways that Sisters in Shape functions as grassroots activism, Cassandra immediately calls attention to the gym as a racially inflected space—an uncomfortable racial zone—a characterization that she then uses to emphasize the importance of Sisters in Shape as an institutional presence at 12th Street Gym: "You can't walk into any other gym and see an organization . . . white women can walk in and they have a network just by virtue of the fact that they're white."

She thinks back to her own experiences working out at a number of gyms over the past three decades to give examples of what she means. At the YMCA, the first gym she joined in the mid-1970s, "there was nobody in that gym who looked like me. Nobody." At times there were black men lifting weights at the gyms she went to, but she still did not see herself reflected in them. Much more recently, she visited a gym in Manayunk, a nearby working-class (but quickly gentrifying) neighborhood of Philadelphia, and found that little had changed over twenty-five years. Given Cassandra's self-confidence, particularly where exercise and weight-lifting are concerned, and her self-identification as a strong, independent black woman, it is no surprise that she has never been intimidated by the lack of people who look like her in these different gyms. She also knows, however, that not all black women share her confidence. In fact, most "need to go in there and find somebody they can identify with. That's what makes this organization and this gym different."

As a more specific example, Cassandra tells me about one of her colleagues, an overweight black woman who joined a gym in a strip mall in the New Jersey suburb of Mt. Laurel. Familiar with Cassandra's deep commitment to her own health and fitness, the woman began complaining to her about her suburban gym almost immediately after joining: "I don't feel like I belong there." In response, Cassandra continually tried to get her colleague to join Sisters in Shape and 12th Street Gym (which happens to be within walking distance of their office and half a block from the high-speed train line to the New Jersey suburbs): "You need a network, you need a sisterhood, you need to join 12th Street Gym. That's what you need to do, you need to, you need to be around the people in Sisters in Shape." In the end, the woman neither joined Sisters in Shape nor returned to the gym she had joined in Mt. Laurel. Instead, she decided to lose weight at home before giving her gym another chance.

With these examples, Cassandra invokes the gym as a site of naturalized racial segregation, at least emotionally, and stresses white women's ease in relation to most black women's discomfort: "White women can walk in and they have a network just by virtue of the fact that they're white . . . there was nobody in that gym that looked like me." Even in this first remark, Cassandra zeroes in on the racially driven contrast between the institutional ("White women . . . have a network just by virtue of the fact that they're white") and the individual ("there was nobody in that gym that looked like me"). Moreover, she offers a range of examples—the YMCA, Main Street Fitness in Manayunk, the anonymous gyms in suburban New Jersey—as well as testimony of her own self-confidence to draw a broader social portrait, to depict a cultural phenomenon where many may see an individual insecurity: "I'm strong enough in myself, that you could put me anywhere and I can figure out, you know, or just give me the weight equipment, but some people need that, they need to go in there and find somebody they can identify with."

For Cassandra, the importance of seeing oneself reflected in the social mirror of a gym is fundamentally related to positive self-esteem and thus fundamental to women's health, and yet the racial components of the problem have been too easily naturalized, dismissed, and articulated with black women's individual behaviors. Even when institutional attempts are made to encourage black women's participation in fitness programs, these social dimensions are frequently overlooked. One research study of a church-based weight-loss and blood pressure control program for black women begins to address the racial and cultural factors contributing to black women's general lack of exercise: "The high receptivity to the exercise component of this project suggests that a lack of convenient opportunities for exercise may be more of a barrier to increasing physical activity among black women than a lack of motivation" (Kumanyika and Charleston 1992: 31). While convenience undoubtedly matters—for instance, Cassandra cites her coworker's commitment to the gym in Mt. Laurel as a matter of convenience that overrides even her extreme discomfort—the "high receptivity" cannot be attributed only to that, especially in a study where everyone is someone a participant can identify with, where everyone is reflected in the social mirror of the workout site.

When Cassandra's coworker complains about her gym—"I don't feel like I belong there"—she cuts to the heart of the problem. Most important, though, is the way that Cassandra responds to this woman's complaint, translating it into a broader theoretical deconstruction of the gym as a raced site, thereby rendering what is most commonly seen to be an individual responsibility as a politicized social issue: "That's because you need a network, you need a sisterhood." Activism exists in the "sisterhood," the network, the transformation of the racially intimidating space into a comfortable social space where black women can see themselves as rightly belonging.

At the same time, Cassandra's colleague's decision to lose weight before returning to the gym suggests that adjunct modes of prejudice such as sizeism and ageism also factor into the gym as a potentially oppressive space, especially if the gym (like the one described earlier) does not feel inherently welcoming or hospitable. Sonja, an inspirational woman in her late 50s, elaborates on Cassandra's theories about the gym as a racially inflected space with her own story of participation in Sisters in Shape and further teases out some of the issues linking self-esteem to the gym with her comments about her sister. Sonja is an impressive woman: an employee in the Philadelphia jails, a grandmother, and an avid (and talented) cook. She was also one of the first Sisters in Shape women I interviewed, and I distinctly remember her smiling broadly as she settled into a cross-legged position on the floor as we made ourselves comfortable in one of the gym's empty workout studios. "I couldn't even do this a few weeks ago," she said, gesturing in slight amazement at the position she had assumed. She has a soft, self-deprecating sense of humor that sometimes becomes a sly, even wicked, one, but both only thinly veil the justifiable pride she feels in having made enormous and successful changes to her eating and exercise habits. A regular participant in all of Saturday's Sisters in Shape fitness classes, Sonja also attends some of Melanie's classes during the week and does cardiovascular workouts early in the mornings before she heads off to work. In addition, she lifts weights with Melanie two to three times a week, depending on her schedule, which fluctuates in accordance with the needs of her mother, who lives with her and for whom she is the primary caretaker.

Sonja also loves to invent new ways of cooking within the Sisters in Shape nutritional guidelines. Indeed, I have never heard anyone describe making an egg-white omelet with such delight. One afternoon she rushed in a few minutes late for our scheduled interview; she had been distracted and delayed by her Sunday postchurch ritual of smoking chicken so she would have tasty, healthy fare readily available during the upcoming week. Though she now loves the challenge of cooking traditional foods in a healthy way and regularly invents new recipes,

Sonja initially found the Sisters in Shape eating plan to be the most difficult of the changes she was trying to make. Her solution was to put a small promotional photo of Melanie on her kitchen table, a constant reminder of both the Sisters in Shape nutritional system and the Sisters in Shape community of which she had become a central part and which would sustain her in her life changes.

As a middle-aged black woman with little previous history of exercise, Sonja confirms Cassandra's sense of the importance of a gym in which black women can see themselves: "That's what I like about it, like nobody says [*imitating a snotty voice*], 'Wow, look at her, why is she here?' I mean [*imitating a nasty voice*], 'She's too old to be in this class.' 'Cause people do that, but they don't see it that way; they like [*sweet voice*], 'Oh come on, you can do it.'" In addition, Sonja also sees herself reflected in and encouraged by women at the gym beyond the Sisters in Shape circle. During one of our interviews, one of the gym's competitive bodybuilders, a black woman in her early to mid-30s, approached Sonja with a catalog for stylish workout clothes—tights and shorts, sports bras, halfshirts. "Here's that catalog I promised you," she said as she handed it to Sonja, who later told me she had commented on the woman's "sharp outfit" during one of her previous visits to the gym. Sonja cited this woman's kindness and enthusiasm as an example of how people in the gym made her feel as though she, too, belonged there (though she also added rather conspiratorially that she doubted she would ever wear any of the clothes featured in the catalog).

The fact that Sonja feels a comfortable sense of belonging at 12th Street Gym also inspired her to try to get her younger sister involved in an exercise program. She describes her sister as "very, very heavy" and "grossly overweight," with such low self-esteem that Sonja cannot imagine even getting her to wear a pair of exercise pants. Nonetheless, she truly believes that if her sister would come to the gym just once, she might see herself reflected in some of the other extremely overweight women who are exercising and participating in Sisters in Shape. Imagining what she would like to say to her sister, Sonja begins, "But you can come because it's all right, because everybody . . . ." Though she trails off before completing her thought, her earlier comments offer some insight as to how she might have finished the sentence (". . . is so nice/welcoming/accepting/safe/familiar"?).

Through these stories and comments, Sonja implies a contrast between her experiences with Sisters in Shape at 12th Street Gym and her experiences at other gyms where she has not felt as comfortable, where people may have thought her too old or wondered aloud what she was doing there. Thus, Sonja not only provides details that complement Cassandra's more general theories regarding the importance of social identification and support, but she also extends Cassandra's discourse on race and gym culture to include other modes of oppression such as ageism and sizeism. In so doing, Sonja begins to elaborate some of the other institutional barriers to black women's exercise, and she draws on her own experiences with age discrimination to reiterate the ways that the institutional is too frequently misread as the personal: "Nobody says, like, 'Wow, look at her, why is she here?' I mean, 'She's too old to be in this class.' *'Cause people do that*" (my emphasis). By speaking aloud what she imagines to be people's questions ("why is she here?") and comments ("she's too old to be in this class") about her participation in gym culture, Sonja clearly acknowledges the judgment she perceives as an individual, older black woman. But, like Cassandra, she uses these hypothetical (or perhaps overheard in other settings) comments as a foil against which to highlight Sisters in Shape as an organizational structure that dismantles these oppressions not only in talk but in action as well.

Sonja's own experiences with Sisters in Shape do not specifically link self-esteem and positive body valuation with the gym as literal and symbolic space, but when she turns to her sister's case she makes this connection explicit. Sonja's specific reference to her sister's low self-esteem as perhaps the greatest barrier to her participating in an exercise program in a gym exemplifies the tragic cycle put into play when institutional and individual aspects of body size, self-esteem, race, and other modes of oppression intersect. As a "grossly overweight" black woman, Sonja's sister is unlikely to feel comfortable in a gym, even one with a relatively high black population; the institutional culture of most gyms reinforces individual tendencies to avoid such spaces for those who do not meet the dominant cultural ideals, particularly white heteronormative ideals. Thus, while the individual and the institutional collaborate in maintaining such cycles, the individual most frequently bears the responsibility for having a body outside the dominant cultural norms.

As Sonja makes clear, however, Sisters in Shape provides an alternative ("if she could come and see some of the other women that are really heavy . . . and that are tryin'"). Indeed, over the course of my work with Sisters in Shape, several very overweight and obese women did participate in the organization. Yet, in the end, few of these women have stayed with Sisters in Shape, a fact that seems to suggest that even under ideal gym contexts providing racial, age, and gender identification, body size and self-esteem (together with the possible traumas underlying their obesity) may be overriding factors for those too far outside the cultural norm. For most others, however, Sisters in Shape transforms the space of the gym by creating an alternative social mirror—one in which black women of varying shapes, sizes, and ages can first see themselves and then see themselves making change on personal as well as social levels. At the same time, narratives like Sonja's and Cassandra's alter the dominant discursive fields surrounding black women's self-esteem, body valuation, exercise, and health by pointing out the fact that getting black women into a gym or an exercise program is not simply a matter of personal motivation but rather a much broader problem of institutional oppressions.

Health Information: Reconsidering Self-Esteem in the Contexts of Race and Responsibility

By intervening in the dominant discourses that position health and fitness as wholly individual responsibilities, the Sisters in Shape women call attention to the larger social bases of health and wellness as well as to the ways that race informs and structures such hegemonic beliefs. While the gym offers a specific site for critiquing the institutional oppressions that sustain these mythologies of individual responsibility for health and fitness, the Sisters in Shape women extend this critique, moving beyond the space of the gym to consider the ways that general health information is also influenced by institutional systems and traditions of racism.

In one instance, Toni, a social worker in her late 30s, alters my question about health information and exercise in African American communities by referring instead to an unnamed study of the differences between black women's and white women's attitudes toward their bodies, thus making explicit the relationship between overall wellness and self-esteem. In so doing, she (re)contextualizes black women's supposedly greater body esteem by suggesting that such attitudes and their negative health consequences emerge from a lack of proper health information, a lack she attributes to a broadly racist culture. After summarizing the general findings of the study, which were reported in a popular magazine or newspaper article—the main thrust of which was that black women feel more comfortable about their bodies than do white women, even when their bodies fall outside medical and insurance health standards (i.e., when they are overweight and obese)—Toni immediately points out the ways that this higher body valuation among black women points to a lack of education about specific health concerns such as hypertension and diabetes. Most significantly, however, Toni does not ascribe this poor health knowledge to the failure on the part of individual women but rather to historical oppression and contemporary institutionalized racism: "I think that for a long time, when you talkin' about African American culture, it goes back to, I don't know, maybe slavery time and the way that, you know, we were taught to eat by bein' given scraps from pigs. I mean, yeah, so I think that it was never, uh, intended for us to be focused on health issues, you know what I'm sayin'?" Toni then goes on to discuss the ways that Sisters in Shape intervenes in a racist social history wherein black women (and African Americans generally) were never intended to have access to crucial health information (a point made painfully clear through the Tuskegee syphilis study, a study that still resonates in African American resistance to white public health efforts).[4]

By essentially reframing my question and offering the example of this article comparing African American and European American women's body satisfaction, Toni not only shifts the focus of my initial question but also significantly recasts the issues at stake in these broader cultural discussions of race and self-esteem. She immediately and powerfully calls out the myth of a potential cultural misunderstanding or a simple cultural difference when she responds to this study by saying, "I think that right there that shows that there was a lack of information about the health issues." While Toni may at first seem to identify the "lack of information about the health issues" as a reason for black women's apparently greater body satisfaction, it becomes clear that she is making a much more radical critique, not of the shaky foundation on which black women's greater level of comfort with themselves rests but rather of the very questions framing the research on race and self-esteem. In following up on her own observation about how this study shows a "lack of information about the health issues" with a specific list of health problems that disproportionately affect black women, Toni implicitly redefines the researchers' concerns—how black and white women feel about their bodies—as superficial when compared to the health statistics of black women.

Perhaps even more telling is the way Toni rearticulates black women's health concerns with slavery. In this discursive move, she uses slavery as both a real and a symbolic source of institutionalized racism and oppression to make absolutely clear her point that black women are not at fault for any lack of information about the health issues. In fact, racism accounts for the skewed (and detrimental) emphasis on body image instead of body health at the core of these cultural debates about race and body satisfaction, a point that Toni articulates explicitly when she moves into the passive voice to describe the roots of African American eating practices: "We were taught to eat by bein' given scraps from pigs." For Toni, this discursive construction emphasizes the larger social and institutional dimensions of racism that have affected and continue to impact black women's health over time. As she makes clear in her pointed conclusion to this initial response, a long legacy of institutional racism has been devastating for black people's health: "I think it was never, uh, intended for us to be focused on health issues."

Ultimately, Toni seems to suggest that concerns over the racial dimensions of women's body satisfaction, the very terms of the research, simply divert attention from the most crucial health issues for black women. Thus, while body-image issues may be one of the most significant health concerns for white women (white women seem historically to have had far higher levels of eating disorders such as anorexia and bulimia, though one study suggests that such differences across ethnicities are diminishing),[5] Toni forces us to disarticulate these concerns as universal women's health priorities. In this way, she begins to address her own sad observation that "we've been measured by somebody else's standard for too long" and to effectively reframe issues of race, body, and self-esteem by (re)centering the discussion on the terms most important for black women's health.

In a related example, Sonja also posits responsibility for health information as a social, cultural, and/or medical concern, though she does
not so drastically refocus the terms of the discussion to call attention to a
problematic framing of black women's health priorities via discourses of
self-esteem and body valuation. In a discursive move that is almost the
opposite of Toni's, Sonja begins with an assessment of her own body—
her rounded stomach (though "not pokin' out beyond [her] bustline"),
the fit of her T-shirt, the way a double-breasted suit now fits her—to
convey a sense of how Sisters in Shape has attracted her for "the long
haul" in teaching her a whole new way of healthy living. She compares
her experiences with Sisters in Shape to other attempts she has made
to lose weight in the past and claims that with previous diets she was
impatient, wanting instant results, measuring herself and her health by
the scale, concerned about dropping dress sizes as quickly as possible.
With Sisters in Shape, on the other hand, Sonja tells me she does not
care how long it takes her to get in shape because she is already healthier
and she plans to stay that way.

In describing her past experiences with dieting and weight loss,
Sonja remarks, "See, I'm not interested, like I used to be, 'Oh, let me
see if I can lose ten, fifteen, twenty pounds,' but really I never cared
about, I wasn't informed enough to know that I should not just lose
weight, I should be pursuin' good health." In moving from the active
voice of "really I never cared about" to the passive construction of "I
wasn't informed enough to know that I should not just lose weight, I
should be pursuin' good health," Sonja reimagines health as a collective effort, and in this sense, her move from active *caring* to the passive
being informed challenges the dominant social understanding of health
as an individual responsibility based on a neoliberal model of capitalist
consumption. In contending not only that she did not care enough but,
more importantly, that she was not informed enough, Sonja suggests
that others—medical workers, weight-loss programs, popular media—
also have a responsibility in overall health education as opposed to diet
(mis)education, and, as a result, she calls attention to the overabun-
dance of diet and weight-loss information in contrast to the paucity
of health information related to body size, weight, and overall health.
Thus, though she and Toni begin from very different discursive positions, both revise hegemonic discourses about black women's bodies to

make explicit the ways that medical ideologies and institutional racisms are often projected onto individual bodies as personal shortcomings.

Body Valuation from the Inside Out: Altering the Body Beautiful

In discussing overall health and medical test results, Cassandra and Melanie establish new priorities—health over appearance—for defining the beautiful black body and, in the process, also redefine self-esteem so that it corresponds directly to a woman's feeling *as* her body and not her feeling *about* her body. This new emphasis on bodily health and the embodied feelings associated with such health completely disrupts the dominant academic and popular discourses concerning race, body, and self-esteem. Cassandra's and Melanie's pride in their own good health, as measured by their own feelings and by biomedical standards, does more than just intervene in these hegemonic discourses, however. Their discussion, replete with examples of specific health indicators, introduces a new model for black women's self-esteem and positive body valuation, one with implications that extend far beyond the body as linked to size, shape, and weight.

Cassandra introduces these topics as she, Melanie, and I are talking (on tape) while waiting for several other Sisters in Shape members to join us for a larger group interview. "You know what's more important to me than how I look?" she asks as an introduction to the topic she wants to address: "How I feel." Both Cassandra and Melanie then proceed to describe how good they feel in ways that remind us of the failure of language to capture embodied feeling with any accuracy; rather, their enthusiasms must oscillate between general proclamations of feeling good and extralinguistic exultations such as "Whooo!" and "Yeah!" until they move to concrete examples of how "feeling good" translates into bodily health: no more headaches, no more stomachaches, no more constipation, and no more premenstrual syndrome or menstrual cramps, for starters. To further validate their subjective understandings of their bodies as "healthy," they also offer medical measures, as Cassandra does in describing a recent checkup with her doctor: "I'm a forty-three-year old African American female with a cholesterol level of sixty. 'Hey now,' the doctor told me, 'sixty? What are you doin'?

Whatever it is, keep it up.' That's a good thing, good blood health." Such descriptions of bodily health—from their own assessments and those offered by medical tests and doctors—not only elaborate what it may mean to "feel good" but also serve as a sharp contrast to a preoccupation, even among many Sisters in Shape members, at least initially, with the external body, what Cassandra calls the "physical, vanity part." Both she and Melanie acknowledge the role that appearance and the physical body play in first attracting women to Sisters in Shape, but they also work against the idea that Sisters in Shape is primarily about weight loss, a point Melanie makes emphatically: "Exactly! . . . Your approach has to be more than just the appearance, like you said, you have to think about the fact that you want to be healthy and you want to live as long as you can."

Cassandra's opening question and ready answer—"You know what's more important to me than how I look? How I feel"—immediately establishes the primacy of feeling good and being healthy in her understanding of what constitutes a beautiful black body. She then follows up her quick response to what she values more than looking good with an extensive riff on how she feels, on the importance of feeling good: "Whooo! I love the feel. I feel good," and later, "That's the thing I like, I like the energy level," and again, "that feelin' you know, that's the thing." From the concrete increase in energy level and overall good feeling to the unspeakable joy ("Whooo!"), Cassandra continually focuses on how she feels so as to capture the unspeakable "Whooo!" that joins the physical to the emotional and the spiritual. In this way, she substantially redefines self-esteem—traditionally, how one feels psychologically about oneself—in a way that necessarily involves psychological *and* bodily feelings.

For Cassandra, looks, the mark of the outside body, seem like simple rhetorical foils against which to highlight her enthusiasm for the importance of feeling good: "I mean, people get into this like, 'You slippin' into those smaller sizes,' that down the road, but that feelin', you know, that's the thing. I think people need to get concentrated on that instead of all that physical, vanity part." And yet, this seemingly incidental discursive move points to a much larger deconstruction of the importance of the body's physical appearance to women's self-esteem. By continually circling back to how she feels as opposed to how she looks, Cassandra rearticulates the cultural logics that yoke women's self-esteem to psychological body satisfaction. Even when I suggest to Cassandra and Melanie that people are motivated to join Sisters in Shape by their desire to change their physical appearance, Cassandra uses that as another opportunity to shift the discursive ground. This deconstructive turn is further articulated in the second half of this conversation, when she and Melanie begin to exchange health reports.

Cassandra's and Melanie's rearticulation of the beautiful body as the healthy body also intervenes in the popular and academic discourses on black women's self-esteem. While self-esteem and body valuation research seems to home in on mental health as the key sign of self-esteem with respect to body satisfaction, Cassandra and Melanie resist this singular focus by integrating self-esteem—what they continually refer to as *feeling*—with physical, psychological, and spiritual health and well-being. Moreover, such a reconceptualization also establishes new priorities premised on the idea that how black women feel *as* their bodies is at least as important as how they feel *about* their bodies. Given black women's dire health statistics, Cassandra's and Melanie's emphasis on an integrated health model of self-esteem is an important discursive activism that introduces a new framework for black women's health praxis.

Rearticulating Self-Esteem: Beyond Body Weight, Shape, and Size

The Sisters in Shape discourses on self-esteem and body (dis)satisfaction suggest that black women's greater body satisfaction and greater self-esteem are myths of both fantasy and fault, myths born of the long-standing ways that black women's bodies have been simultaneously articulated with both resistance and excess. These mythologies have deep currents throughout the research literature and the popular media and are well represented by the articles in *Essence* and the *New York Times* discussed earlier. That is, on the one hand, black women's supposed greater body esteem is celebrated as a healthy resistance to white heteronormative body ideals and a welcome rejection of mediated body expectations: "Black women may be buffered from negative mental health consequences of weight concern and embodied femininity by socially critical and skeptical attitudes. . . . Black women may use a social critique of ethnicity and gender to protect themselves from the negative implications of pursuing largely unattainable ideals" (Bay-Cheng et al. 2002: 42). On the other hand, black women's higher body esteem is cited as one of the cultural causes of high levels of obesity and poor health statistics for black women: "For some Black women, a positive body image may be an expression of denial of psychological and physical health problems, such as obesity and compulsive eating" (Lovejoy 2001: 255).

To be sure, researchers and writers rarely endorse only one of these perspectives but rather tend to prioritize one or the other, most often without fully considering the social and cultural contexts of interlocking systems of racism, sexism, and classism that necessarily structure these issues.[6] At the same time, I do not mean to imply that these readings have no relation to the lived experiences of black women as they work to sustain healthy body attitudes in the midst of a mediated society with sexist and racist underpinnings. What I mean to highlight, rather, is that the academic and popular discourses of black women's supposed higher body satisfaction and self-esteem tend toward limited interpretations that simultaneously frame and constrain the conversation. Limiting research questions to assumptions of difference as opposed to the more complex *meanings* of specific differences (such as those developed by Becky Thompson [1994] and Tamara Beauboeuf-Lafontant [2009]) has been a long-term strategy for social scientific scholarship, as Collins points out in her analysis of the role that black women have played as objects of knowledge in sociological investigation (1998: 103). Thus, as Bay-Cheng and colleagues make clear in their review of the literature, some researchers have argued that "the needs of Black women in the domains of weight concern and disordered eating are being overlooked" (2002: 37).

Not surprisingly, many of the Sisters in Shape women's comments confirm the fact that black women's needs are not being met by the terms of the studies intended to investigate the racial aspects of weight concern and self-esteem. By delineating a context-specific black feminist standpoint, the Sisters in Shape women situate themselves as a collective response to what they see as an incredibly common discourse of low (or lacking) self-esteem among the black women they know. Thus, aside from contesting the most basic findings at the heart of the studies demonstrating that black women have greater body satisfaction than do white women, the Sisters in Shape women's conversations continue to diverge sharply from the hegemonic discourses on race, the body, and self-esteem, thereby forcing new options for understanding black women's self-esteem issues as related to their bodies. Together, their examples emphasize the ways that the Sisters in Shape women reorient the terms of the discussion on self-esteem, race, weight, body shape, and body size to draw out the concerns that are most important to them, concerns often overlooked entirely in the research and popular literatures.

Throughout our general discussions about Sisters in Shape, Melanie extends issues of self-esteem beyond the body and draws out the relationship that self-esteem has to the whole person. She immediately joins the physical with the spiritual and the emotional—"this physical fitness thing that they're doing, it translates into other areas of their lives, spiritually and emotionally"—in a move that firmly emphasizes the complex aspects of a person as opposed to the singular pursuit of bodily perfection often associated with exercise programs. In so doing, Melanie shifts the grounds of the discourse and opens up different possibilities for understanding how race, body issues, and self-esteem affect black women.

In one example, Melanie tells me about the fifty-five-year-old wife of a local minister, a woman who fully understood herself in relation to the role she thought she had to play as the well-known man's wife. Not only did she perform a range of social duties for the parishioners, but she also did all of the domestic labor for her husband—who "happens to be pretty lazy when he's not on the pulpit"—and his mother, who lives with them. Upholding the image and expectations of a "minister's wife," she essentially cared for everyone but herself; between the needs and desires of the people at church and the needs and demands of the people at home, she rarely had a moment of her own. This woman joined Sisters in Shape after reading the *Daily News* article, began participating in some of the general Sisters in Shape activities, and even started weight training with Melanie. A few weeks later, she was refusing to wait on her husband and mother-in-law "hand and foot" as she had for her entire married life up to that point. In fact, according to Melanie, she claims that Sisters in Shape had such an effect on her life that when the minister and his mother asked her to do something ordinary, to get them something, she responded with a new attitude: "You have legs, why don't you get it yourself?" Taking a stand for herself, she let them know that she was no longer there to serve them: "Hey, I am not here to serve you. I am your wife, I am your daughter-in-law, but you have two legs and you're askin' me to do things that you can do with no problem at all."

Through this story, Melanie underscores the relationship that Sisters in Shape posits between self-esteem and empowerment. By drawing out the logic whereby women's participation in a health and fitness program increases their self-esteem so that they no longer stand for oppressive (and socially sanctioned) behaviors, Melanie rescripts the issues at stake in the broader considerations of race, body, and self-esteem. Whereas the research and popular literature seem continually to circle back to the individual—whether through an emphasis on mental health problems, an emphasis on individual body satisfaction, or an emphasis on eating disorders—Melanie forces a consideration of self-esteem as related to the social as well as to the individual. Increased self-esteem has the capacity to alter the social body and the individual body, as women such as the "minister's wife" question accepted social dynamics of gender hierarchy and traditions of filial piety (or filial *in-law* piety, as the case may be and often is). Here, then, Melanie begins to expose the structures supporting the current emphases in much of the research. If the greatest, gravest concerns (and expectations for solutions, therapies, and remedies) for white women with respect to body image and self-esteem are bounded by the individual and are singularly focused on how an individual woman copes with body dissatisfaction (e.g., Allan, Mayo, and Michel 1993; Bay-Cheng et al. 2002; Lovejoy 2001; Bowen, Tomoyasu, and Cauce 1991; Gray, Ford, and Kelly 1987; and Rand and Kuldah 1990), then such dictates will necessarily determine the course of investigation. Melanie's insistence on self-esteem as linking the physical, emotional, and social offers a glimpse beyond the dominant structures.

In somewhat similar fashion, two other examples extend issues of self-esteem beyond the body and body (dis)satisfaction to suggest important ways that black women's individual body concerns affect a wide range of social and emotional behaviors and attitudes. In her mid-20s and approximately eighty pounds overweight, LaTanya was one of the first Sisters in Shape members I met after the frantic organizational rebirth of Sisters in Shape. She was also one of the most enthusiastic members of the group, and she often fantasized aloud about where Sisters in Shape was headed—exercise and diet books, appearances on *Oprah*, health education classes at black colleges, a fast-moving grass-roots movement for and by black women. She, too, had learned about Sisters in Shape through the article in the *Daily News*, though it was her father who first saw the article and called her away from her work and her "half-eaten hoagie" to read it. He even offered to pay for her to join Sisters in Shape and, eventually, to train with Melanie three times a week. Excited and impatient for change after talking with Melanie on the phone about a month before the symposium, LaTanya took an enormous calendar, circled the date of the symposium, and began crossing off the days with a fat red marker, much as a child would count down to Christmas.

Taking her father up on his generous offer, she was one of the first women from the symposium to submit a personal trainer request form. On it she wrote, "I'm sick and tired of being sick and tired. I just want this weight off. I really want to lose."[7] Committed from the start, LaTanya worked hard and began to see some results. "Enthusiastic" does not do justice to her attitude. Melanie remembers one instance when LaTanya called her on the phone, really excited, and asked to meet her a bit earlier than their scheduled training session because she had something to show her. When Melanie arrived at the gym, LaTanya was wearing a dress, and she said, "Look, look," as she gestured at her body in the dress, which fit her beautifully, no longer tight and bulging in spots as it had been only a short time before.

The first time I talked with LaTanya, I asked her to tell me her story. In response, she chose to tell me what Sisters in Shape had done for her up to that point. She began by telling me that "everybody says I'm glowing," that she is very perky, has really high energy, and is caring and friendly, all accurate self-perceptions as far as I could tell from my thoroughly enjoyable interactions with her. What surprised me was when, after detailing these positive attributes, she said: "It's like my whole person has really really really changed." Changed from what, I wondered (and asked), since I simply could not imagine LaTanya any other way. "I was very moody; I was very mean," she replied. "I was very nasty,

I was very short. I never knew why, I had a attitude, I was mad against the world; it was like I was takin' on the world at all times."

Another woman, Bev, was also really angry, though more at herself than at the world. In her mid-40s and already a partner in a prestigious law firm, Bev seemed almost desperate when I first met her. Clearly smart and accomplished in her professional life, she seemed defeated by her body. Melanie remembers some of their first interactions as marked by Bev's anger: "She walked in and she was like [*disgusted voice, imitating Bev*], 'I'm so *disgusted* [*long and drawn-out*] with myself; I can't *believe* I let myself get like this,' and she was just mad." Almost the polar opposite of LaTanya, Bev stayed mad for her first week or two training with Melanie and participating in Sisters in Shape events and classes; she would come to the gym and work out hard, but she was angry the whole time, huffing and puffing in exaggeration to express some of her resistance. About six weeks after joining Sisters in Shape, Bev's whole attitude had changed. She had become, in Melanie's words, "a beautiful, accepting person who's ready to do what she needs to do." She had also lost about fifteen pounds in that time, and people she knew were commenting on her physical changes. In addition, she claims that her higher body valuation also increased her sense of empowerment and her ability "to deal" with virtually all other parts of her life, including some that she believed to be potentially destructive.

While these accounts from LaTanya and Bev are slightly less explicit in articulating a connection between increased self-esteem and overall personal liberation and well-being, they still provide examples that continue to reorient the dominant ways of understanding race, body (dis)satisfaction, and self-esteem. At the same time, LaTanya's and Bev's narrative accounts of their experiences resonate with both Becky Thompson's and Tamara Beauboeuf-Lafontant's findings that black women may turn to food as a protection against both social and personal oppressions and traumas. Both LaTanya and Bev suggest that their anger was a signal of low self-esteem, and though neither of them names her low self-esteem outright (as many of the Sisters in Shape women do when they describe their motivations for joining the organization), their memories and narrative self-imitations imply as much. LaTanya's scribbled plea ("I'm sick and tired of being sick and tired. I just want this weight off") is echoed in Bev's claims of self-disgust ("I'm so *disgusted* with myself" and "I can't believe I let myself get like this"). For both women, their body dissatisfaction carries over into other parts of their lives and erupts in the form of anger, resentment, and, as LaTanya characterizes it, a "mad[ness] against the world." Indeed, LaTanya's own portrait of herself as an angry young woman suggests some of the ways that self-esteem has broad social and individual implications; her feeling "mad against the world" and her sense of having to "[take] on the world at all times" point to the ways that she was overwhelmed by her own negative body esteem (and low self-esteem generally) while also calling attention to the social effects of body dissatisfaction among black women. The fact that anger surfaces several times in these interviews as an expression of body dissatisfaction suggests *not* that body concerns and self-esteem are not significant issues for black women but rather that most researchers have misread (or misconceptualized in the asking) the contexts in which black women are voicing concerns about their bodies and about their health in relation to their bodies.

Like LaTanya, Bev was "very angry," "MAD," and "pissed"—aspects of her general attitude that disappeared as she began to feel "just wonderful about herself" and empowered. According to Melanie, as Bev transitioned from "disgusted" and "pissed" at herself to "empowered," she also made changes in other parts of her life. As Melanie describes it, Bev's new sense of herself carries over into other, more challenging parts of her life: "She's feelin' just wonderful about herself, and it's translatin' into other parts of her life because she's got other things goin' on that can potentially set her back if she let it." This connection that Melanie forges between Bev's higher body esteem and her ability to handle other trying aspects of her life is a significant means of challenging the standard discourse on race, body, and self-esteem that focuses on self-esteem as linked directly (and in the research, solely) to body weight, shape, and size. Here, Melanie, Bev, and LaTanya extend the parameters of the discourse by insisting on the ways that higher body esteem translates into other, non-body-related facets of a woman's life. This interventionist discourse calls into question the overemphasis on body and replaces it with a concern for the whole person: "They, their self-esteem goes up. It just improves every part of their being." Here, Melanie equates the women with their self-esteem, beginning her sentence with a reference to the Sisters in Shape women but immediately substituting "their self-esteem" as the subject of the sentence, a rephrasing that belies her truest beliefs that self-esteem not only is a part of the person but also constitutes the person.

New Bodies of Knowledge: The Politics of a Sisters in Shape Standpoint

The Sisters in Shape women's everyday conversations and organizational discourses specify some of the ways that issues of black women's self-esteem are integrated into broader social concerns. By altering, shifting, and reorienting the dominant discourses to prioritize their own experiences as sources of information, the Sisters in Shape women produce new bodies of knowledge capable of explaining their own everyday lived realities while establishing new paradigms for black women's bodily visibility. The Sisters in Shape women's rearticulations intervene in hegemonic academic and popular accounts of black women's bodies and black women's beliefs about their bodies, accounts that begin with and continue to reinscribe their assumed inherent difference from a white normativity.

Through these discursive practices, the Sisters in Shape women also highlight the significance of a collective identity based on multiple and shifting selves for generating a context-specific standpoint that fosters new critical theory, political change, and social justice. Such a context-specific standpoint challenges Collins's reliance on a stable group identity at the center of her intersectional standpoint theory even as it adds a new dimension to her claim that black feminist thought is one way of sustaining an oppositional consciousness and critique: "For Black feminist thought, remaining oppositional involves challenging the constructs, paradigms, and epistemologies of bodies of knowledge that have more power, authority, and/or legitimacy than Black feminist thought" (1998: 88). As the Sisters in Shape women make clear, such an oppositional consciousness resists hegemonic interpellations and dominant representations and insists on new epistemologies that might enable a productive identity politics.

This oppositional consciousness also grounds the Sisters in Shape women's epistemic status as *black women*, what Mohanty would refer to as their "realist" identity, specifically these black women whose experiences give rise to a new body of knowledge about black women's body esteem. While the more general category of *black women* builds on a constructionist foundation and underscores the ways that social identities are produced when ideological formations are mapped onto material bodies in historically constrained and nonarbitrary ways, the Sisters in Shape "realist" identity and context-specific standpoint suggest that there is also always at least some room for self-definition and self-determination in collective rearticulations (as the group similarly demonstrates through its performances of multiple black womanhoods and its resistance to dominant interpellations discussed in the previous chapter). The Sisters in Shape women's ability to organize around a context-specific standpoint and to assert an oppositional consciousness illustrates the undeniable potential of identity politics for both social recognition and new epistemological claims.

At the same time, while such theories of identity may allow for diversity within the group, they also tend to preclude an articulation of too much diversity. Rather, identity groups necessarily rely on a collective interpretation of experience according to the group's dominant self-definitions, a tendency that complicates the group's self-determination by overgeneralizing the bases of their social and political claims to justice. As an example, the Sisters in Shape women's focus on anger as an index of low self-esteem forecloses other potential readings of anger as a justifiable response to being a black woman in a racist and sexist culture. Though many feminists have read anger in this collective way (see Scheman 1980; Spelman 1989; and Holmes 2004 for detailed discussions), and such a reading may also contribute to a context-specific, shifting standpoint, LaTanya and Bev clearly invoke their anger in a way that further consolidates Sisters in Shape's dominant discourses: as an individually located emotion linked to their low self-esteem, a connection they can overcome through their engagement with Sisters in Shape.

Given the Sisters in Shape women's impulse to foreground the social dimensions of many different problems—such as the lack of comprehensive health care and health education, the gym as a raced and gendered site, and black men's supposed love of big black women—LaTanya's and Bev's emphasis on anger as individually located is particularly striking. The group's discursive coherence around the issue of anger raises the question of how alternative understandings of LaTanya's and Bev's claims might affect the potential effectiveness of group-based claims to social justice. Thus, while this chapter has detailed the capacity of a context-specific and embodied Sisters in Shape standpoint to make use of discourses of self-esteem in order to intervene in dominant epistemologies of gender, race, and health and to generate new bodies of knowledge, the next chapter attends to the potential downsides of a feminist standpoint theory that depends on such discourses for its claims to social recognition and action.

5 / Rearticulating Feminist
  Identity Politics

As I have been arguing throughout *Body Language*, the Sisters in Shape women's attention to the body—the deeply corporeal nature of the experiences, discourses, and performances through which they produce their shifting and multiple identities—opens up alternative ways of conceptualizing some of the questions about identity and identity politics at the center of feminist theory. Foregrounding the embodied dimensions of the Sisters in Shape women's subjectivities as fundamental to any understanding of their politicized identity helps mediate the falsely dichotomous impulses that tend to structure such questions. Along these lines, the previous three chapters have offered examples of the Sisters in Shape women's particular contributions to debates about experience, performativity, and standpoint in relation to collective consciousness, political agency, and social change. Insofar as these theoretical debates lend important insight into processes of identity formation and the emergence of political consciousness, they also highlight the most pressing question for feminist identity theory: whether identity-based claims to social change and social justice are viable modes of political action.

While many theorists have argued against identity groups as agents of political change, Wendy Brown offers one of the most compelling critiques in her theorization of the relationship between identity-based claims to justice and ressentiment from her well-known article "Wounded Attachments" (1993). Drawing on Nietzsche's definition of ressentiment as "the triumph of the weak *as* weak" (quoted in W. Brown 1993: 400), what she herself terms "the moralizing revenge of the power-less" (1993: 400), Brown is careful to point out that ressentiment is not so much an ongoing sense of victimization as a logic driving political claims about exclusion through recourse to pain and suffering. For her, politicized identity is both a product of and a reaction to the conditions of late modernity wherein suffering becomes morally virtuous. In an effort to displace this suffering, politicized identity invests in its own subjection, thereby unintentionally subverting attempts to achieve its goals. According to Brown, ressentiment prevents identity groups from accessing the rights they seek both because such a group's ontological grounding in injustice ensures that it remain forever injured in the eyes of the state and because its very existence as a group depends on the continuation of that injury.

Simultaneously bound to the injurious history that produced it and "reproach[ful] of the present that embodies that history," politicized identity ironically forecloses a desire for an alternate future, a future that "triumphs over this pain" (W. Brown 1993: 406). Against this prob-lematic whereby the loss of futurity is essentially refigured in an identity politics structured by a desire for normative inclusion and recognition, Brown seeks to recover a desire that exists prior to the initial wounding, thus reopening a possible future. To this end, she advocates "supplant-ing the language of 'I am' . . . with the language of reflexive 'wanting'" (1993: 407) as a way of disrupting "I am" as "a resolution of desire into fixed and sovereign identity" (1993: 407). Unlike "I am," "I want" cannot mark a fixed position but rather reveals a desire for something to come, something other than a longing for inclusion of the sort structured by late modernity. For Brown, this desire for an alternative future enables an identity outside a constitutive wounding, an identity not already fore-closed at the moment of its inception.

I focus here on Brown's "Wounded Attachments" because her nuanced argument against identity politics has come to epitomize the "anti-identity" position[1] and because her emphasis on ressentiment, together with her opening up of an alternative future for an identity premised on desire, raises questions of particular relevance to the Sisters in Shape women's identity politics. As detailed in the previous three chapters, the Sisters in Shape women's collective identity formation and their interventions into dominant epistemologies depend on collective discourses of self-esteem that seem to counter the anger fundamental to ressentiment. Unlike the logic of self-esteem that seems to underlie many, if not all, identitarian movements in the insistence that people be recognized for who they are *now* as opposed to who they must become in order to be legitimated by the state and society (a form of self-esteem consistent with ressentiment), the Sisters in Shape discourses of self-esteem tend to offer an alternative way of understanding the feelings that might be interpreted as anger were they to emerge in a different social context.

Such discourses depend on a largely unquestioned, taken-for-granted, and positive understanding of self-esteem, however. For the Sisters in Shape women, the wholehearted embrace of self-esteem may create blind spots with regard to some structural oppressions, including those they critique elsewhere. Thus, I begin by pushing against the Sisters in Shape women's unquestioning commitment to self-esteem as a way of further exploring the overall effectiveness of identity politics in light of Brown's claims about ressentiment's powerful logic. I then consider the ways that the Sisters in Shape women's discussions of self-esteem are wrapped up in the past, in the time before Sisters in Shape, as well as how they gesture toward the future, how they are entangled in the promise of a self and a body to come. Through such constant becomings, the Sisters in Shape women encourage a more extensive investigation into the possibility of an alternative politics as suggested by Brown in her theorization of an identity based on desire and an open futurity. I conclude by focusing on the ways that such a future orientation proves critical to the Sisters in Shape women's rearticulation of feminist identity politics.

Subjects of Self-Esteem

At the end of the previous chapter, I suggested that Sisters in Shape's foundational discourses of "improved self-esteem" encourage an understanding of LaTanya's and Bev's initial anger as an index of their lack of self-esteem before joining Sisters in Shape, even though their anger may just as reasonably be a response to their specific experiences of being black women in a racist and sexist culture. For instance, as an obese, young, black woman, LaTanya's being "moody," "mean," "nasty," and "short"; having "a attitude," being "mad against the world"; and feeling like she was "takin' on the world at all times" may just as well represent feelings that derive from the social marginalization and invisibility accompanying her particular subject position. Labeling such feelings "anger" as well as understanding and claiming them as a legitimate response to structural oppression are expected outcomes of second-wave feminist politicization of the sort that often occurred in consciousness-raising groups (e.g., Scheman 1980; Spelman 1989; and Holmes 2004). While second-wave feminists helped women interpret their feelings as anger, directed toward patriarchal institutions and individual behaviors, they frequently remained ambivalent about such expressions because of the normative gender proscriptions against them (Scheman 1980; Holmes 2004); these gender norms also had serious implications for feminists' willingness to engage in conflict and to address the anger that sometimes arose among them in their efforts to communicate and organize across differences such as race, class, and sexuality (Holmes 2004; Lorde 1984). Nonetheless, anger has been a fundamental aspect of feminist political critique.

For the women of Sisters in Shape, those feelings not only originate in the individual but also depend on the individual for their resolution, albeit through the help of the group's practices. In positing two different ways of understanding LaTanya's and Bev's feelings and experiences, I do not mean to suggest that one is more valid or relevant than the other. Rather, the dramatically different meanings given to similar feelings within the context of second-wave feminism and contemporary Sisters in Shape discourses simply reiterate the fact that feelings and experiences are generally made intelligible and come to be articulated through the social contexts in which they are enmeshed. For second-wave feminist consciousness-raising groups, articulating such feelings with anger is an explicitly political act, whereas for the Sisters in Shape women the articulation of such feelings with an initially low self-esteem to be improved through participation in the group makes it a largely individual concern.

The fact that what some may perceive to be the Sisters in Shape women's anger and frustration is first given meaning and then addressed through the idiom of self-esteem is hardly surprising given the widespread attention to self-esteem in contemporary American culture. Though early references to "self-esteem" date back to the fourteenth century (Stephenson 2004: 17), the current American preoccupation with it is generally attributed to the 1970s and the 1980s, when aging countercultural activists began to struggle with the disappointment of unrealized revolutionary social change, self-help practitioners began to appear regularly on daytime talk shows, and educational and political leaders began to associate an extensive range of social ills with their perpetrators' low self-esteem (Rapping 1996; Hewitt 1998; Stephenson 2004; and Ward 1996). Popular theories and beliefs about self-esteem grow out of late nineteenth- and early twentieth-century writings on self-psychology and mid-twentieth-century psychological and sociological research into "self-concept" as related to individual behaviors and social problems (Hewitt 1998; Stephenson 2004; see Ward 1996 for an extensive overview of the development and popularization of the concept of self-esteem). As is the case with the women of Sisters in Shape, few people doubt the value of self-esteem as described in popular discourses despite the fact that at least two extensive academic reviews have determined that there is no causal relationship between self-esteem and the long list of the qualities, behaviors, and benefits that supposedly accrue from it (Hewitt 1998; Rapping 1996).[2] In essence, the widely held popular beliefs about, and faith in, self-esteem continue to override the research findings, a testament to its enormous cultural appeal.

One of the obvious problems in popular discourses of self-esteem and in the Sisters in Shape discourses is the term's widespread use and tendency to stand in for many different feelings, emotions, and psychological states. While people often assume "self-esteem" to mean "self-regard" or "self-worth," in everyday contexts it frequently stands in for "happiness" and "success" or, when lacking, for "depression" (Hewitt 1998: xiii, 139–140); in the Sisters in Shape context, it takes on these connotations as well as others related to spirituality, overall health, and emotional well-being. This slipperiness—together with self-esteem's popular perception as a panacea for everything from poor math and reading skills to substance abuse, sexual violence, and tyrannical political leadership—evacuates much of the specificity from the Sisters in Shape women's collective discourses as well as from their personal accounts of their experiences with the group. Even more problematic, perhaps, is the implicit individualization of structural problems fostered by a self-esteem paradigm. Such a paradigm locates the source of social problems and the responsibility for their solutions within the individual, thereby neglecting more politicized accounts of power, difference, historical context, and institutional oppressions that may also be relevant, particularly for those who occupy marginalized subject positions.

The Sisters in Shape women's emphasis on self-esteem as an individual concern may seem especially remarkable considering their focus on the social dimensions of everyday problems and institutional oppressions in a wide range of other contexts. However, as many social critics have argued, the pursuit of overall health and well-being has become a key aspect of subject formation in contemporary, neoliberal societies that cultivate individualist ideologies with respect to holistic health and general happiness (e.g., Crawford 1980, 2006; Lupton 1995; Galvin 2002; McGregor 2001; Dworkin and Wachs 2009; and Ferguson 2007). In a society where attaining and maintaining health are "qualities that define the self" (Crawford 2006: 402), it is not surprising that the Sisters in Shape women internalize the extensive cultural messaging imploring each of us—through the idioms of rationality, normativity, morality, and mortality—to take responsibility for our own health, broadly defined.

Unlike many of the other hegemonic messages that the Sisters in Shape women contest, resist, and rearticulate, the cultural association between health and identity allows for a certain degree of control, an ability to influence one's own health and happiness within a racist and sexist society that—in many ways—creates and sustains health disparities. This understanding obviously begins with the neoliberal ideology of individualism, but it suggests some of the appeal for the Sisters in Shape women. That is, just as some women may find an otherwise unavailable control in anorexia, bulimia, and other modes of disordered eating, so too may the Sisters in Shape women find a similar control in their pursuit of health and positive self-esteem.

Solutions to the host of personal ailments that emerge when social problems are located within the individual and associated with a lack of self-esteem find ready expression in the closely related self-help and recovery movements. Elayne Rapping has mapped the extensive scope and ideological reach of what she calls the "culture of recovery" through her analysis of recovery movement discourses in popular media— particularly self-help "gurus" on daytime television and mainstream self-help books and magazine articles—and through her ethnographic research into several different self-help and recovery groups based on the Alcoholics Anonymous twelve-step model (1996). Although Sisters in Shape neither functions as nor identifies itself with the recovery movement, many of the group members' claims about its influence on their self-esteem are steeped in the language and ideas of the culture of recovery. As an example, in LaTanya's account of always being "mad against the world" before joining Sisters in Shape, she moves seamlessly from her description of feeling like she was "takin' on the world at all times" to the language of recovery when she talks about Sisters in Shape's effect on her life: "Now, I find myself at peace. I'm at peace right now. I do a lot more prayer. I talk to myself as much as I possibly can, and I feel as though I live every day as if it was my last, and that is my motto, 'I live every day as if it is my last.'"

LaTanya's peace, her prayer, and her personal motto all correspond with and even echo the Christian underpinnings and social ideologies of contemporary recovery programs, particularly those based on the twelve-step model. What she appropriates as "her" motto—"to live each day as if it is my last"—calls to mind not only the twelve-step dictum to "take one day at a time" but also the general practice of drawing on such inspirational quotes and phrases, circulated in recovery groups and self-help books, as a way of daily reminding oneself of one's values and goals (Rapping 1996: 115, 134). In drawing on the language of the recovery movement, LaTanya not only testifies to its cultural power and pervasiveness but also affirms and shares its prioritization of the self as the site and source of change.

Like LaTanya, several other Sisters in Shape women highlight the importance of prioritizing, attending to, and loving the self if one is to make lasting personal changes, thus emphasizing the way that recovery and self-esteem are inextricably linked. In one instance, Miriam shifts the focus of a group conversation about other people's negative reactions to how much money she spends to train with Sisters in Shape by emphasizing the importance of loving oneself: "You see, that's why I think it's the focus on the self . . . do you love yourself, 'cause you take on a whole new aspect, 'this is about me and this is not about you,' this is not about family or relationships . . . this is all about you." Like a self-help expert, Miriam reminds the other Sisters in Shape women that "this is all about you" and not about families or other relationships, a central tenet of the recovery movement generally and groups like Co-Dependents Anonymous in particular (Rapping 1996: 115).

In a different discussion about how people go about making dramatic lifestyle changes like the ones she has made, Charlie says almost the same thing about loving oneself: "The first thing, you have to love yourself, if you love yourself that much, then you wanna take care of yourself and you need to take care of yourself and takin' care of yourself means, 'Okay, I know I need to get some exercise.'" For both Charlie and Miriam, loving oneself is fairly mundane. It involves exercising with Sisters in Shape, not participating in an "addiction" recovery group where people share the details of their lives, past and present, or "get up and shout 'Me! Me! Me! I matter!' to group applause," as Rapping describes in an extreme example (1996: 116). Thus, what seems to matter most for the Sisters in Shape women is not so much the recovery paradigm as its fundamental attention to improving and sustaining one's self-esteem as the primary mechanism for change.

Nonetheless, LaTanya, Miriam, and Charlie all (perhaps unintentionally) discursively associate Sisters in Shape with a recovery group, an association that Melanie likewise fosters in characterizing the Sisters in Shape "program" as a journey: "This program is designed to last forever; it's a journey, it's not a destination. You never, it's not a program where you start, you do it for X period of time, and you stop." Thus, despite the fact that Sisters in Shape is not a recovery group, the idea that "it's a journey, it's not a destination" suggests otherwise in the popular cultural vocabulary. According to Rapping, the driving logic of the recovery movement is that "one is born, or becomes, an addict. . . . One hits bottom; one sees the light; one works one's program, every day for the rest of one's life, and is, from then on, in 'recovery'" (1996: 9). Melanie's description of the Sisters in Shape "program" clearly corresponds with Rapping's description of recovery programs, a point reiterated when

Melanie recounts for me her advice to a long-standing Sisters in Shape member who put herself on a juice diet in an attempt to lose weight more quickly:

> And I told [her], I said, "Stop looking for solutions, you got this plan, that plan, that plan, that you're askin' so many people so many things, you're getting all confused as to what you should be doing. You have to believe in what your plan is; if you don't believe in your plan, find another plan and work it, but you got one that works, you see everybody doin' it, working it."

Although Melanie's admonishments to this woman are expressed in the language of self-help and recovery, her advice to the woman to "work" the plan she has or find another one grants the woman more agency than the typical twelve-step model, wherein people begin by admitting that they have no power over their addictions. Thus, even as Melanie's language converges with that of the recovery movement, the underlying principles are different in certain fundamental ways.

What the Sisters in Shape women likely find most relevant about the recovery movement, what they take up in their "recovery talk," is the attention to the self as the site of productive change and the broader group support for making such changes and attending to the self. As mentioned earlier, Sisters in Shape workshops and publications are replete with calls for black women to stop putting everybody else first, to take care of themselves if only to better care for others; within this context, the recovery movement's foundational idea that individual and social well-being are rooted in love and care of the self lends credence to the Sisters in Shape women's choices and permits them to challenge the expectation that they must live up to the myth of the strong black superwoman. "Loving oneself" is an especially important concept for women who have been bombarded with the message that they should be caring for everybody else before themselves. In alluding to the fundamental changes necessary to overcome addiction, the language of recovery also resonates with the Sisters in Shape belief that the group is teaching women to make ongoing lifestyle changes and acknowledges the difficulty of those changes and the ways that such dramatic shifts frequently challenge their relationships to family, friends, and the various communities of which they are a part.

Even though those "in recovery" tend to focus on the personal implications of social injustices rather than engage in political critique, Rapping argues that the culture of recovery has been shaped by many of the political practices, methodologies, and gains of the second-wave feminist movement. More specifically, for Rapping, feminism and the recovery movement are linked in at least two important ways. First, she contends that women's disappointment in feminism's inability to achieve the sweeping social transformations that seemed possible during the height of the 1960s progressive social movements has been so profound that women have largely given up faith in political and structural change, believing instead that their discontent has both its sources and its solutions in the self and in interpersonal relations. At the same time, Rapping argues, in increasing many women's educational and employment opportunities, shifting gender and family expectations, and giving name and meaning to such violent phenomena as date rape, sexual abuse, and domestic violence, second-wave feminism fundamentally altered our cultural ideals for intimate and family relationships in ways that may still differ for women and men and/or in ways that may be difficult to achieve given the everyday realities of modern capitalist society.

According to Rapping, the self and its relations have become a focal point for all of the expectations and disappointments inspired by the second-wave feminist movement, and one of the primary reasons why so many participants in the self-help movement are women has to do with the fact that "the recovery movement, in taking feminism more seriously than the current Left, offers women something which we cannot so easily dismiss because we have nothing, at the moment, to replace it" (1996: 11). In keeping with Rapping's claims about the gendered appeal of the culture of recovery, the Sisters in Shape women seem to find a certain empowerment in addressing injustices through collective discourses of the self.

As previously mentioned, self-esteem features prominently within recovery culture, and Rapping provides a cogent and cutting account of the depoliticizing impulses and the "logical slippages" at the center of popular and policy attempts to improve self-esteem as a way of solving structural inequalities and social problems. While Rapping's criticisms refer specifically to the California Task Force on Self-Esteem's publication *Toward a State of Esteem* (California State Department of Education 1990), she extrapolates from that analysis to critique the self-esteem movement as a whole. Perhaps most significant, she also underscores the self-esteem movement's lack of attention to "power relations in a materially unequal world" (Rapping 1996: 177), its turning away from what feminists accepted as the need for "bloody struggles over power and money" to bring about radical social transformation (177).

As a paradigmatic example of the feminist shift from a focus on explicit political critique and mobilization to a focus on self-esteem, Gloria Steinem's *The Revolution from Within* (1992) draws on the teachings of the recovery and self-esteem movements to suggest ways that she and others might heal their wounded inner children so as to live more satisfying lives and, in her case, to better accomplish her political work. Although Rapping acknowledges Steinem's efforts to situate concerns about self-esteem and childhood injuries within an explicitly political context, she nonetheless astutely reads *The Revolution from Within* as a "[move] away from a clear sense of what the social problems are for us and why they have proved so hard to eradicate" (Rapping 1996: 179). As both Steinem and Rapping make clear, no longer is the personal political; rather, they argue—one implicitly, the other explicitly—that the personal has replaced the political.

The culture of recovery, facilitated and sustained by both the self-esteem movement and the feminist movement, is full of paradoxes and contradictions. For Rapping, it is simultaneously political and apolitical, wrapped up with the goals of feminist social change even as it moves away from broader structural concerns and diminishes the political urgency of claims to justice. Thus it lends insight into Sisters in Shape's complex relationship to self-esteem. On the one hand, the Sisters in Shape women's tendency to cast their experiences in the language of recovery, with its emphasis on the self and self-esteem, exemplifies Rapping's point that addressing the *effects* of social injustice as if they were *causes* originating in the self depoliticizes claims for justice and forces the individual to bear responsibility for any redress. On the other hand, as a project explicitly by and for black women, Sisters in Shape differs dramatically from the mostly white, upper-middle-class "women's" recovery groups that Rapping attended and from the assumed audience for mainstream books and the self-help experts on daytime television. Within the contexts of Rapping's fieldwork and her research focus on the mainstream culture of recovery, her description of the self of the recovery movement as "a spiritual and biological, but *not* a social, entity" (1996: 161) makes perfect sense. The women of Sisters in Shape, however, are inherently social entities, perhaps not so much by choice as by their overdetermined subject positions as black women. Their coming together as such—the fact of their collective identity, even consolidated through discourses of self-esteem—reiterates the already social and political nature of their group. Indeed, this is what makes their relationship to self-esteem so complex. In foregrounding the power of self-esteem in their collective discourses, the Sisters in Shape women focus inward even as their group identity connects them to broader social concerns and disrupts dominant cultural beliefs about them.

Always already imbricated in identity politics, the question is not so much whether Sisters in Shape is political but whether the group's emphasis on black women's improved self-esteem is an effective strategy for change, especially as a way of resisting ressentiment's controlling logic. Despite Sisters in Shape's politicized, *collective* relationship to self-esteem and the interventions into hegemonic epistemologies and dominant representations of black women and their bodies that it enables, the group's overriding discursive and embodied practical reliance on the *individual* as the locus of change has an ironically similar effect to ressentiment in terms of diminishing the potential for a transformative politics based on identity. However, as I have been arguing throughout *Body Language*, the Sisters in Shape women's identity politics are also always embodied and corporeal, and the centrality of the body to their collective praxis might still open up alternatives to a politics of identity structured by ressentiment.

The Body to Come

Above all else, Sisters in Shape is about self-transformation—of the body and the individual—through exercise, nutrition, and community, and the Sisters in Shape women have improved their health status in a number of different ways. Given black women's disproportionately high rates of heart disease, adult-onset diabetes, and obesity (U.S. Department of Health and Human Services, Agency for Healthcare Research and Quality 2009; Grady 2010), the Sisters in Shape women's weight loss and its effects on their cholesterol levels and blood pressure, together with their commitment to exercise and their understanding of nutrition, are critical interventions. In examples such as Cassandra's low cholesterol levels and Justine's healthy weight gain during her pregnancy, the Sisters in Shape women offer an alternative picture of black women's health in the contemporary United States.

At the same time, the self-transformations of the Sisters in Shape women are also about a perpetual becoming, about the desire and drive for another body, another self, an idealization always located somewhere in the future. For these women, the group's core practices, its exercise regimens and nutritional guidelines, are invested with the promise of a body to come, whether in terms of shape, size, strength, health factors, or overall feel, as is the case for many people preoccupied with exercise and/or restricted eating. Although the desire for a body to come is so naturalized among the Sisters in Shape women that it need not be spoken, it is nonetheless a common topic of discussion and one of the factors that core members see as central for bringing new women into the group. In describing the educational impact of Sisters in Shape's aerobics demonstrations at health fairs, for instance, Melanie recalls one audience member's desire to be among the women onstage as a motivation for her eventually joining the group: "She specifically told me she was very inspired, and she said, 'Boy, I look forward to the day when I can get up there and be one of those Sisters in Shape.'"

LaTanya expresses the same sentiment in a much more personal manner in response to one of my questions about how the women present see themselves influencing others through their participation with Sisters in Shape:

My main part of Sisters in Shape is waiting to do what Denise [Murphy] did when I first met Denise and the fact that it was a year ago when she started. Now I'm waiting for the big year, redoing the favor, "I started with Melanie a year ago and look at me now and my role in Sisters in Shape is X, Y, and Z, and just because you're whatever, do not make age a reason for you to start, stop makin' excuses. [**Melanie:** Yeah.] There's a reason what brought you to the symposium that day that means you're interested, you wanna make a change, make a change tonight, and introduce yourself to Melanie and that's how we get the balls rolling."

In this example, LaTanya imagines her future self sharing her story as a way of encouraging other women to make the changes she presumes she will have made ("and look at me now") after her first year with Sisters in Shape. Indeed, she goes so far as to preview exactly what she will say in a year's time, clearly having imagined herself in that future context many times before. That textual detail, along with the fact that LaTanya's future story as she recounts it has not yet fully transpired, underscores the taken-for-granted nature of her future orientation. None of the Sisters in Shape women present during this interview think twice about the fact that after only eight weeks, LaTanya is already rehearsing what she will say in talking about the changes she has made to her body ten months into the future. For LaTanya, the desire for a future body also extends beyond her anticipating how she may inspire others; rather, her commitment to a body to come seems to structure her whole perspective on life. In another example, she tells me a story about a man who whistled at her as she was walking down the street. She turned to him and hollered back, "Not today; this time next year we can talk but not right now, I'm on a mission."

While LaTanya's description of her prospective motivational speech and her response to the man who whistled at her illustrate well the ways that a desire for a body to come is quickly and easily integrated into her understanding of Sisters in Shape, group members more typically imagine their future bodies through references to their current ones. In a series of conversations spanning several different interviews, Sonja touches on the myriad ways that the Sisters in Shape women conceive their future bodies. During our first interview, she described her excitement about joining Sisters in Shape with a general approach to her future body, telling me that she "started lookin' forward to getting to that little person that's inside of me, thought he'd [*sic*] come out again, and I started gettin' positive thoughts about that." A bit later in the same interview, she offers a much more specific desire when she says, "I'm lookin' forward to bein' able to get my leg up straight," a desire she echoes in another interview as she anticipates her cardiovascular progress: "I'm lookin' forward to the time that, uh, maybe four or five months down the road, where I will be able to just, really just do a half hour right along with the class without feelin' like I'm gonna pass out from exhaustion."[3]

At other times, Sonja sounds a lot more like LaTanya as she imagines her body several months, one year, ten years, even twenty years into the future:

"I can't wait to see myself this time next year."

"I can't wait to see myself in December" (said in July).

"I'm not lookin' to suddenly be a twelve in three months or four months or five months; I know I'm gonna get there."

"In ten years, she [Melanie] gonna show me off as a sixty-seven-year-old woman, and I'm gonna be sixty-seven and I'm gonna be all that."

"When I get seventy-five, I'm gonna still be wearing heels. I'm not gonna need a cane, because I'm gonna have strong muscles and if I keep doin' weight trainin' stuff . . . I'm gonna be, I may look seventy-five from the face, but the body will not."

Sonja's obvious investment in her body to come as represented by these sequential visions underscores the perpetual nature of such desire.[4] Whether imagined through corporeal measures such as being able to lift her leg or through external measures such as fitting into a size 12 or being "all that" when she is sixty-seven, Sonja's comments about the various stages of her future body exemplify the dominant Sisters in Shape discourse of their program being a "journey" as opposed to a "destination," and for her, this series of bodies is like a set of markers along the way, each one promising progress toward the next.

The metaphor of Sisters in Shape as a journey, with its implication of lifelong participation and a future destination, is especially apt for conveying the never-ending chain of desire implicit in always imagining oneself as a future body. While a constant and continuous longing for a body to come may seem to suggest a dissatisfaction with one's present self, the Sisters in Shape women's faith in their improved and improving self-esteem seems to counter that idea. For them, self-esteem conflates present and future such that the Sisters in Shape women's feeling good about themselves now, their being "at peace," and their loving themselves ironically enables and sustains the desire for a future body, one marked by better health, greater ability, and a more ideal size and shape.

In focusing on the future as opposed to the injurious past—the "negative energy that has gotten us to the point where we were" in LaTanya's words, the being "taught to eat by bein' given scraps from pigs" in Toni's example, and echoed in Allison's point that frying with lard "goes so far back in our culture [because] we had to like make do with whatever was there"—the Sisters in Shape women gesture toward what Franz Fanon saw as the freedom possible in the future, a future in which he was not "a prisoner of history" (quoted in Kruks 2001: 103), neither looking to the "great African cultures of the past" nor "focusing on resentment over past injuries and demands for reparations" for a black identity (Kruks 2001: 103). Though Kruks goes on to critique Fanon's understanding of freedom as too radically individual—she cites his claim to be his "own foundation" (103)—and thus too detached from the social and historical realities with which the individual is always bound, the Sisters in Shape women's specific future orientation, underpinned by desire for a different (corpo)reality, recuperates some of the hope inherent in Fanon's freedom.

For the Sisters in Shape women, the hope animating the continual movement toward a future body, reflected in the logic and language of "I want," is fundamental to transforming their "I am." In fact, this endless desire, this perpetual becoming, defines Sisters in Shape and, in keeping with Brown's theoretical exploration of the political implications of such a shift, helps generate a different type of identity on which to stake their claims for recognition and social justice. A Sisters in Shape identity predicated on a desire for a future self, a body to come, insists on a corporeal subjectivity and highlights its grounding in the inextricably linked—in Möbius strip fashion—experiences as determined by both language and embodiment. An identity forever in motion, forever resisting fixity, likewise holds together the fluid and multiple selves evoked by Sisters in Shape's ongoing identity performances and attests to the power of the social and political interventions made possible through such embodied and shifting subjectivities, the microinterventions into the politics of the everyday and the broader interventions into dominant epistemologies and representations. Wrapped up in the historical and social circumstances of their raced and gendered subjectivities even as they produce themselves through a future desire, the Sisters in Shape women bring to life Stuart Hall's understanding of identity formation as "using the resources of history, language and culture in the process of becoming rather than being" (1996: 4). Insofar as Sisters in Shape's collective identity depends on an endless desire for a body to come, it "[recovers] the more expansive moments in the genealogy of identity formation" (W. Brown 1993: 407–408), and the Sisters in Shape women can alter the possibilities for identity politics by coming together as a group outside the controlling logic of ressentiment.

Rearticulating Feminist Identity Politics

When the *Philadelphia Daily News* article that changed the Sisters in Shape world first appeared, I had been training with Melanie for about a year. We lifted weights together twice a week, I took her exercise classes, and she taught me principles of nutrition relevant to the fitness regimen I had undertaken. During our sessions together, we also spent a lot of time talking about our personal and work lives. When the *Daily News* article came out, I witnessed its impact firsthand, and when the calls kept coming, I had the opportunity to help Melanie think through the various options she was considering for meeting the sudden, even overwhelming, demand for information, service, and help. In this way, I have been a part of Sisters in Shape from the beginning of its transformation, helping Melanie plan and organize the first symposium and having an intimate, embodied familiarity with the exercise and nutrition practices at the center of the Sisters in Shape program. Thus, I have simultaneously always been something of a Sisters in Shape insider and, as an Asian American woman, an obvious outsider, and this duality has necessarily informed my research.

Because I am a half-Chinese, half-Japanese third- and fourth-generation Asian American raised in an upper-middle-class California suburb, my racialization and my gendering have been dramatically different from those of the women of Sisters in Shape. Even the expectations and idealizations I had for my body were distinct from those I heard expressed during my many conversations with the Sisters in Shape women, and it was soon readily apparent that our notions of what constituted a "great body"—at least in terms of size and shape—were also substantially different. While I aspired to look like a teenage boy with minimal musculature and few curves, they were trying to look like Melanie, with her well-defined, big, full muscles. Our many differences were, and are, such that I am sure I have at times misunderstood aspects of what the Sisters in Shape women were telling me, what they may have been trying to tell me by politely (and indirectly) returning to subjects I was ready to leave or insistently digressing from topics I refused to let go. In some cases, after countless close readings of our conversations, I believe I have begun to understand their efforts; in other instances, in the moment and in my interpretations, I am sure I have not. My own identity formation and personal desires make it likely that I have projected my experiences with race, ethnicity, gender, and embodiment onto the Sisters in Shape women's personal narratives and insights even as I have tried to understand them on their own terms—tried to avoid romanticizing them, condescending to them, or simply misrepresenting them. Of course, to acknowledge the complex politics of qualitative research is not to abandon all hope for some meaning grounded in our coming together. Any interaction with an "other" is subject to miscommunication and misunderstanding and is run through with differential power; I thus do not want to overfetishize the power of the researcher—my power—as constitutive of their being as I try to account for our differences and possible failures to communicate.

Nor do I want to suggest that the different ways that the Sisters in Shape women and I are raced and gendered make any identification between us impossible. As women who have exercised together, women with a lasting faith in a future body, albeit a differently imagined one, we have shared certain embodied practices and experiences even as we are shaped by a range of differently subjectifying discourses and powers. As Kruks has argued, such embodied experiences and ways of knowing can inspire a feminist identity politics that accounts for women's differences while allowing for the possibility of broader coalitional politics that exceed the limits of what she calls an "epistemology of provenance" (2001: 21–22), the limiting tendency of identity groups to stake claims based on the distinctiveness of their particular experiences. For Kruks, it is through affect and the sentient "pre-conceptual ways of 'knowing' through our bodies (bodies that are both anatomically sexed and deeply gendered)" that we "[feel]-with others" (163) and, through that corporeally grounded feeling-with, that we might come to political identification and solidarity.

Kruks's examples of "feeling-with" are largely drawn from her volunteer work in a battered women's shelter and relate to the physical pain of domestic abuse. Within this context, she is careful to distinguish her theorization of "feeling-with" as a basis for political articulation and solidarity across difference from simply assuming another's pain. As Kruks describes it, her pain at seeing a woman's battered face is physical but not of the same type as the woman's own pain: "In a certain doubling of embodied awareness, my body was a locus of pain that was distinct from hers, and yet my body was also connected to hers since my (dissimilar) pain was engendered by feeling-with hers" (2001: 166). According to Kruks, this painful knowing in a similarly sexed and gendered body moves one to take up the cause of another and, in so doing, to politicize that cause. She similarly argues that our corporeal knowing—our "gut feelings" about injustice, for instance—are often the first stimulus to action, that which moves us to solidarity with an "other" (145).

Extending Kruks's examples beyond the context of pain and injustice, I want to suggest that shared embodied experiences may likewise motivate solidarity and contribute to coalitions based on identifications and understandings other than those structured by historical and social determinants. Over the course of my research, the Sisters in Shape women and I often seemed to share such embodied sensations as pleasure, laughter, muscle burn, sweat, and fatigue. Sometimes we whooped together, a vocal release of energy, a sign of joy beyond the strictures of language; sometimes we grunted in exhaustion or pleasurable pain, and sometimes we were silent together, still nonetheless joined in bodily awareness and deep corporeal attention. While we may have experienced our exercising differently, we were united in our concentration on our bodies, their movements, and their corporeal sensations. That we often responded to our experiences in similar expressions that escaped language—whooping, laughing, grunting—suggests that in many instances we were indeed "feeling-with" each other.

In a similar case, Deidre Sklar draws on her own ethnographic field-work and corporeal participation in two different religious rituals that fall outside her personal background to argue that such shared embodied experiences lend insight into cultural knowledges that would otherwise remain inaccessible: "I had discovered that to 'move with' people whose experience I was trying to understand was a way to also 'feel with' them, providing an opening into the kind of cultural knowledge that is not available through words or observation alone" (1994: 11). In addition to their methodological importance, Sklar's corporeal experiences partici-pating in the women's section of a Hasidic *Purimspiel* in Brooklyn and in the annual Tortugas fiesta honoring Our Lady of Guadalupe reiterate the ways that differently located people can join each other in social solidarity, and perhaps even shared cultural knowledge, through Kruks's "doubling of embodied awareness."

While the implications of such embodied identification and solidar-ity are obviously significant for my own ethnographic relationship to the women of Sisters in Shape, they are much more profound for what they suggest about Sisters in Shape's rearticulation of feminist identity politics. As an exercise program specifically for black women, Sisters in Shape's collective identity is repeatedly enacted in and through their raced and gendered bodies in ways that also open the group to the pos-sibility of sharing embodied experiences with differently positioned oth-ers even as they continue to maintain their own specific, ever-shifting identities.[5] The possibilities for connecting across difference, of build-ing on the "doubling of embodied awareness," are further consolidated through Sisters in Shape's future orientation, by the group's perpetual becoming and endless desire for a body to come since such a desire underpins the embodied experiences that enable such connections.

Through their collective praxis, the women of Sisters in Shape co-create new bodies and new discourses, thereby intervening in dominant representations of black women and black women's bodies and contrib-uting to a different material (corpo)reality, not just for themselves but for other women as well. In the end, their distinctive combination of embodied practices and discursive productions helps reconcile many of the tensions implicit in feminist theories of identity, and their lived realities call attention to the fact that experience, subjectivity, agency, and political change are simultaneously deeply embodied and discursively constructed, simultaneously language and corporeal experience. Through their embodied subjectivities, premised on both a corporeal knowing and a longing for a body to come, the Sisters in Shape women create a collective political identity structured by something other than a wounding, a political identity not foreclosed by the controlling logic of ressentiment but open to potential solidarities that might help usher in a truly alternative politics.

Notes

Chapter 1

1. See Alcoff et al. 2006 for a detailed discussion of this position.

2. See Kruks 2001: 107–128 for an extensive consideration of this assumption.

3. I discuss what this may mean in the context of self-esteem discourses in more detail in Chapter 5.

4. These stereotypes derive from racist legacies and popular representations. From the era of slavery, "mammy" refers to the faithful "house servant," a sexless provider and nurturer, while "Jezebel" refers to the seductress with an insatiable sexual appetite and "Sapphire" references an aggressive, mouthy, emasculating character from the *Amos and Andy Show* of the 1950s.

5. Gala True, Ph.D., consulting medical ethicist at Einstein Medical Centers, personal communication.

6. I address the dynamics of gym space and social (in)visibility in more detail in Chapter 5.

7. See Shaw et al. 2004; Counihan 1999; Bordo 1985, 1993; Chernin 1981, 1985; Brumberg 1990; Fallon, Katz, and Wooley 1994; and Gordon 1990 for good overviews and historical perspectives.

8. All names and identifying details have been changed, with the exception of Melanie's and those of the early Sisters in Shape cofounders, Kathy Tillery and Carethia Thomas. In addition, Denise Murphy is referred to by name in regard to the *Philadelphia Daily News* article but not in the remainder of the ethnography.

9. Here, Sisters in Shape is largely consistent with the research on class, gender, and exercise. See, for instance, Shinew et al. 1995 and Floyd et al. 1994 for the differences between black and white participation in exercise among self-identified poor and working-class interviewees. Their studies find that among self-identified poor and working-class people, black women were least likely to exercise when compared with black men, white men, and white women of similar class backgrounds. See also Powell et al. 2006 for a discussion of how structural inequalities related to socioeconomic status, such as the lack of facilities for physical activity and exercise, contribute to lower rates of participation in physical activity among people with lower socioeconomic status.

10. I discuss my status as both insider and outsider in greater detail in Chapter 5, where I situate myself as an Asian American woman and a researcher in relationship to the Sisters in Shape women as a way of thinking through the possibilities that Sonia Kruks (2001) imagines for a coalitional politics based in affective connections.

11. Though I cite Laclau and Mouffe 1985 here because of the extent of the authors' consideration of articulation, Laclau's work on articulation predates this coauthored work.

12. Collins reads *articulation* as having close affinities to intersectionality, and her critique emerges as she attempts to underscore intersectionality's greater relevance for her particular project. I want to emphasize my own difference from this position, as I do not find the same affinities between theories of articulation and intersectionality. In fact, they strike me as operating in distinctly different registers: articulation characterizes unnatural linkages made natural, whereas intersectionality tends to describe intentional points of convergence useful for analysis as well as action.

13. As Nelson writes, "Fluidarity is a practice and a theory of identity-information, aware of its own investments, the pleasures of intervention, and the erotics of relational subject-making. It is historically specific and knows that it is very hard to give up solid bodies, clear-cut enemies and friends, but that this may be the most responsible way to approach the current conjuncture in Guatemala" (1999: 37).

14. James Clifford, comments made at a graduate student conference on psychoanalysis, University of California Santa Cruz, May 19, 2007.

15. While Butler continues to develop her theory of gender performance in her later work, most notably "Melancholy Gender/Refused Identification" ([1995] 1997), I first take up feminist engagements with her early work because of its extensive and ongoing influence in a range of different disciplines.

Chapter 2

1. Here, Kruks engages the phenomenology of Merleau-Ponty, as have other feminists positing sentient knowledges in the body; see, for instance,

Bigwood 1991; Grosz 1993, 1994; Marshall 1996; I. Young 1980; Studlar 1990; and Fisher 2000.

2. Both Miriam and Toni characterized themselves as "depressed," but these characterizations seem to draw on a more vernacular (as opposed to clinical) understanding of depression. At the same time, both women also seemed to exhibit signs of depression like social withdrawal, lack of interest in various work and social activities, and fatigue. For more on black women and depression, see Warren 1997; Barbee 1992; Siegel, Yancey, and McCarthy 2000; Boyd 1999; Mitchell and Herring 1998; and Brown and Keith 2003.

3. See, for instance, Ann DuCille's "The Occult of True Black Womanhood: Critical Demeanor and Black Feminist Studies" (1994) and Tricia Rose's *Longing to Tell* (2003) for more extensive discussions of the romanticization of black women and black women's groups as "naturally" strong and resistant.

4. See, for instance, Jacques Lacan's "God and the Jouissance of Woman" (1985) for a relevant theoretical psychoanalytic perspective.

Chapter 3

1. See Sara Salih (2004: 1–4) for a discussion of the intentionality and political underpinnings of Butler's tendency toward difficult theoretical formulations that defy easy interpretation and understanding.

2. While Butler's and even Beauvoir's theories of gender subjectivity refer to everyday, commonsense, taken-for-granted performances of gender, driven by hegemonic definitions of both gender and sex, they also apply to these interviews in which Sisters in Shape members seem to be consciously playing with the tensions that exist between commonsense and revised notions of race and gender as related to black women.

3. See, for instance, L. Brown and Mussell 1984; Mintz and DuBois 2002; Williams-Forson 2006; Neustadt 1992; Shortridge and Shortridge 1998; Gabaccia 1998; Pilcher 1998; and Counihan and Van Esterik 1997.

4. These beliefs about the strong black woman are prevalent in both hegemonic and African American discourses, although black women may respond to them differently depending on their source. For instance, some of the women in Beauboeuf-Lafontant's study were critical of the oppressive and exploitative aspects of such discourses within a largely white workplace while still internalizing aspects of the myth within their own communities. In addition, I explicitly mark heterosexuality in this sentence because of the gendered and sexed expectations within many African American (and other) households. For instance, in her qualitative work interrogating the myth of the strong black woman, Tamara Beauboeuf-Lafontant shares a number of women's narratives of their own or other women's performing in ways that maintain the image of patriarchal dominance within the household (2009: 86–87); similarly, one woman she interviewed suggests that lesbian relationships offer a type of reci-

procity and accommodation not traditionally available in heterosexual relationships (88–89). For more on black sexual politics, see Jacqueline Jones [1985] 2010; Collins 2004; Bambara 1970; Cole and Guy-Sheftall 2003; Lubiano 1992; and hooks 1981.

5. Now, several years after this exchange, I realize that perhaps I was the one not getting it. Listening to our conversation and repeatedly reading the transcripts, I wonder whether my stubbornness was in fact simply cultural ignorance. Maybe I didn't understand the importance, for these women, of fulfilling the traditional and culturally significant role of caretaker and provider. Moreover, I wonder whether this extended dialogue was, in part, an attempt to educate me, albeit politely.

Chapter 4

1. See, for instance, Allan, Mayo, and Michel 1993 for nursing; Rand and Kuldah 1990 and S. Thompson and Sargent 2000 for medicine and public health; and Bay-Cheng et al. 2002; Flynn 1999; Frisby 2004; C. Hall 1995; Roberts et al. 2006; and Penkal and Kurdek 2007 for psychology.

2. This logic reveals the extensive assumption that thinness automatically correlates with health, and the dominance of this body ideology is reflected in the starting assumptions of much of this comparative work. While obesity is certainly a cofactor in a range of health problems such as heart disease and adult-onset diabetes, some studies also suggest that health and weight may not be so directly linked (see, for instance, Oliver 2006; Kingsbury 2008; and Etheridge 2009). What I want to point out here is the hegemony of the paradigm that equates thinness with health, a naturalized position that marginalizes research studies and personal experiences suggesting otherwise.

3. On the flip side, many women also find bodily and personal control in disordered eating practices such as bingeing, purging, and dieting, particularly in contexts where they may have no other ways of ensuring their bodily autonomy such as childhood sexual abuse and rape (see, for instance, B. Thompson 1994).

4. The Tuskegee syphilis study was a long-term research effort by the U.S. Public Health Service designed to follow the natural development of syphilis among black men, most of whom were rural, extremely poor, and uneducated. None of the men enrolled in the study were told that they had syphilis, and none were offered penicillin once it was determined to be an effective treatment; on the contrary, they were led to believe they were being treated for "bad blood" despite the fact that they were receiving no treatment at all. Conducted between the late 1920s and the early 1970s, the study is now infamous for its lack of ethics. For more detailed accounts, see James Jones 1981 and Reverby 2009.

5. See Shaw et al. 2004 for more detailed information on eating disorders across ethnicities.

6. In my critique of the dominant academic research and popular reporting on the differences between black and white women's self-esteem relative to body weight, shape, and size, I have the opportunity for a much fuller discussion of these issues than the various researchers and authors have in their specific focus on the differences in self-esteem and their consequences for women's mental (and, to a limited degree, physical) health. That said, however, I remain committed to a critique of the ways that these studies and reports seem so often to misread or fall short of understanding black women's self-esteem issues because of their underlying assumptions, rooted in a white, heteronormative epistemology, and the power of those assumptions to structure the research questions and paradigms for interpretation.

7. The phrase "sick and tired of being sick and tired" was first expressed by Fannie Lou Hamer as a "rallying cry" during the 1960s civil rights movement (S. Smith 1995: 14); since then, its use as more generalized black folk speech continues to reference those original associations.

Chapter 5

1. See Susan Bickford's "Anti-Anti-Identity Politics: Feminism, Democracy, and the Complexities of Citizenship" (1997) for a good overview of the "anti-identity politics" and "anti-anti-identity politics" positions.

2. California's attempt to legislate programs to increase people's self-esteem exemplifies this point. The first charge of the state's Task Force to Promote Self-Esteem and Personal and Social Responsibility was to review the research on self-esteem. After an exhaustive review, the task force found that "the associations between self-esteem and its expected consequences are mixed, insignificant, or absent" (quoted in Hewitt 1998: 60). Nonetheless, and despite the dissent of several task force members from the final report, most of the task force members continued to promote self-esteem as a significant remedy for an extensive range of individual and social ills, and the task force sought to reframe the findings so as to bring them more in line with their commonsense faith in the power of self-esteem (Hewitt 1998: 58–61).

3. This comment is characteristic of Sonja's tendency toward exaggeration and self-deprecating humor; when we did this interview, she was already close to keeping up in class and certainly not about to pass out from exhaustion.

4. See Lacan's *Écrits* (2002) for a psychoanalytic perspective on infinite desire.

5. The collective pleasure that spread through Melanie's aerobics classes when the Sisters in Shape women were present offers a minor, but concrete, example that highlights the real possibility of doubled embodied awareness across differences.

References

Alcoff, Linda Martín, Michael Hames-García, Satya P. Mohanty, and Paula M. L. Moya, ed. 2006. *Identity Politics Reconsidered*. New York: Palgrave Macmillan.

Allan, Janet D., Kelly Mayo, and Yvonne Michel. 1993. "Body Size Values of White and Black Women." *Research in Nursing and Health* 16: 323–333.

Anderson, Benedict. 1983. *Imagined Communities: Reflections on the Origin and Spread of Nationalism*. London: Verso.

Angier, Natalie. 2000. "Who Is Fat? It Depends on Culture." *New York Times* (November 7): F1.

Anonymous. 2004. "Eating Disorders Don't Discriminate." *Essence* 35 (June): 36.

Anzaldúa, Gloria. 1987. *Borderlands/La Frontera*. San Francisco: Spinsters/Aunt Lute Foundation.

——. 1990a. "Bridge, Drawbridge, Sandbar or Island, Lesbians-of-Color Haciendas Alianzas." In *Bridges to Power: Women's Multicultural Alliances*, ed. Lisa Albrecht and Rose M. Brewer, 216–231. Philadelphia: New Society.

——, ed. 1990b. *Making Face, Making Soul/Haciendo Caras*. San Francisco: Aunt Lute Foundation.

Baker-Fletcher, Karen. 1998. *Sisters of Dust, Sisters of Spirit: Womanist Wordings on God and Creation*. Minneapolis, Minn.: Augsburg Fortress Press.

Bambara, Toni Cade. 1970. "On the Issue of Roles." In *The Black Woman: An Anthology*, ed. Toni Cade Bambara, 1010–1110. New York: Signet.

Barbee, Evelyn L. 1992. "African American Women and Depression: A Review and Critique of the Literature." *Archives of Psychiatric Nursing* 6 (5): 257–265.

Bay-Cheng, Laina Y., Alyssa N. Zucker, Abigail J. Stewart, and Cynthia S. Pomerleau. 2002. "Linking Femininity, Weight Concern, and Mental Health among Latina, Black, and White Women." *Psychology of Women Quarterly* 26: 36–45.

Beauboeuf-Lafontant, Tamara. 2003. "Strong and Large Black Women? Exploring the Relationships between Deviant Womanhood and Weight." *Gender and Society* 17: 111–121.

———. 2005. "Keeping Up Appearances, Getting Fed Up: The Embodiment of Strength among African American Women." *Meridians* 5: 104–123.

———. 2007. "'You Have to Show Strength': An Exploration of Gender, Race, and Depression." *Gender and Society* 21: 28–51.

———. 2009. *Behind the Mask of the Strong Black Woman: Voice and Embodiment of a Costly Performance.* Philadelphia: Temple University Press.

Bello, Marisol. 1998. "Shape Up, Sisters: Stats: 52% of Black Women Overweight." *Philadelphia Daily News* (March 20): E1.

Bickford, Susan. 1997. "Anti-Anti-Identity Politics: Feminism, Democracy, and the Complexities of Citizenship." *Hypatia* 12 (4): 111–131.

Bigwood, Carol. 1991. "Renaturalizing the Body (with the Help of Merleau-Ponty)." *Hypatia* 6 (3): 54–73.

Bordo, Susan. 1985. "Anorexia Nervosa: Psychopathology as the Crystalization of Culture." *Philosophical Forum* 17: 73–105.

———. 1993. *Unbearable Weight: Feminism, Western Culture, and the Body.* Berkeley: University of California Press.

Bowen, D., N. Tomoyasu, and A. Cauce. 1991. "The Triple Threat: A Discussion of Gender, Class, and Race Differences in Weight." *Women and Health* 17: 123–143.

Boyd, Julia A. 1999. *Can I Get a Witness? Black Women and Depression.* New York: Plume.

Brown, Diane R., and Verna M. Keith, ed. 2003. *In and Out of Our Right Minds: The Mental Health of African American Women.* New York: Columbia University Press.

Brown, Linda Keller, and Kay Mussell. 1984. *Ethnic and Regional Foodways in the United States: The Performance of Group Identity.* Knoxville: University of Tennessee Press.

Brown, Wendy. 1993. "Wounded Attachments." *Political Theory* 21 (3): 390–410.

Brumberg, Joan Jacobs. 1990. *Fasting Girls: The History of Anorexia Nervosa.* New York: New American Library.

Butler, Judith. 1990. *Gender Trouble: Feminism and the Subversion of Identity.* New York: Routledge.

———. 1993. *Bodies That Matter: On the Discursive Limits of "Sex."* New York: Routledge.

———. (1995) 1997. "Melancholy Gender/Refused Identification." In *The Psychic Life of Power: Theories in Subjection*, 132–150. Stanford, Calif.: Stanford University Press.

Cahn, Susan K. 1994. *Coming on Strong: Gender and Sexuality in Twentieth-Century Women's Sport.* New York: Free Press.

California State Department of Education. 1990. *Toward a State of Esteem: The Final Report of the California Task Force to Promote Self-Esteem and Personal and Social Responsibility.* Sacramento: Bureau of Publications, California State Department of Education.

Cannon, Katie G. 1988. *Black Womanist Ethics.* Atlanta, Ga.: Scholars Press.

———. 2006. "Response" to Monica A. Coleman's "Must I Be a Womanist?" *Journal of Feminist Studies in Religion* 22 (1): 96–99.

Captain, Gwendolyn. 1991. "Enter Ladies and Gentlemen of Color: Gender, Sport, and the Ideal of African American Manhood and Womanhood during the Late Nineteenth and Early Twentieth Centuries." *Journal of Sport History* 18 (1): 81–102.

Chernin, Kim. 1981. *The Obsession: Reflections on the Tyranny of Slenderness.* New York: Harper and Row.

———. 1985. *The Hungry Self: Women, Eating, and Identity.* New York: Time Books.

Chirea, Yvonne. 2003. *Black Magic: Religion and the African American Conjuring Tradition.* Berkeley: University of California Press.

Clifford, James. 2001. "Indigenous Articulations." *Contemporary Pacific* 13 (2): 468–490.

Cole, Johnnetta B., and Beverly Guy-Sheftall. 2003. *Gender Talk: The Struggle for Women's Equality in African American Communities.* New York: One World/Ballantine Books.

Coleman, Monica A. 2006. "Must I Be a Womanist?" *Journal of Feminist Studies in Religion* 22 (1): 85–96.

Collins, Patricia Hill. 1991. *Black Feminist Thought.* New York: Routledge.

———. 1996. "What's in a Name? Womanism, Black Feminism, and Beyond." *Black Scholar* 26 (1): 9–17.

———. 1998. *Fighting Words: Black Women and the Search for Justice.* Minneapolis: University of Minnesota Press.

———. 2004. *Black Sexual Politics: African Americans, Gender, and the New Racism.* New York: Routledge.

Counihan, Carole, and Penny Van Esterik. 1997. *Food and Culture: A Reader.* New York: Routledge.

Counihan, Carole M. 1999. *The Anthropology of Food and Body: Gender, Meaning and Power.* New York: Routledge.

Crawford, Robert. 1980. "Healthism and the Medicalization of Everyday Life." *International Journal of Health Services* 10 (3): 365–388.

———. 2006. "Health as a Meaningful Social Practice." *Health: An Interdisciplinary Journal for the Social Study of Health, Illness and Medicine* 10 (4): 401–420.

Crenshaw, Kimberlé. 1991. "Mapping the Margins: Intersectionality, Identity Politics, and Violence against Women of Color." *Stanford Law Review* 43 (6): 1241–1299.

Crenshaw, Kimberlé, Neil Gotanda, Gary Peller, and Kendall Thomas, ed. 1995. *Critical Race Theory: The Key Writings That Formed the Movement.* New York: New Press.

Davis, Angela Y. 1981. *Women, Race, and Class.* New York: Vintage Books.

Derrida, Jacques. (1974) 1997. *Of Grammatology,* trans. Gayatri Spivak. Baltimore: Johns Hopkins University Press.

Dorsey, Allison. 2002. "'White Girls' and 'Strong Black Women': Reflections on a Decade of Teaching Black History at Predominantly White institutions (PWIs)." In *Twenty-first Century Feminist Classrooms: Pedagogies of Identity and Difference,* ed. Amie A. Macdonald and Susan Sanchez-Casal, 203–231. New York: Palgrave Macmillan.

DuCille, Ann. 1994. "The Occult of True Black Womanhood: Critical Demeanor and Black Feminist Studies." *Signs* 19 (3): 591–629.

Duggan, Cheryl A. 2000. *Refiner's Fire: A Religious Engagement with Violence.* Minneapolis, Minn.: Augsburg Fortress Press.

Dumas, Tia Noelle. 2004. *Women of Color in Sport: A Literature Review of the History and Current Status of Women of Color in Intercollegiate Coaching and Athletic Administration.* Thesis, University of Oregon.

Dworkin, Shari L., and Michael A. Messner. 1999. "'Just Do' What? Sport, Bodies, Gender." In *Revisioning Gender,* ed. Myra Marx Ferree, Judith Lorber, and Beth Hess, 341–362. Walnut Creek, Calif.: AltaMira Press.

Dworkin, Shari L., and Faye L. Wachs. 2009. *Body Panic: Gender, Health, and the Selling of Fitness.* New York: New York University Press.

Etheridge, Eric. 2009. "The Thins versus the Fats." *New York Times* (August 2). http://opinionator.blogs.nytimes.com/2009/07/30/the-thins-versus-the-fats/. Accessed August 2, 2009.

Eugene, Toinette M. 1995. "There Is a Balm in Gilead: Black Women and the Black Church as Agents of a Therapeutic Community." *Women and Therapy* 16 (2–3): 55–71.

Fallon, Patricia, Melanie A. Katz, and Susan C. Wooley, ed. 1994. *Feminist Perspectives on Eating Disorders.* New York: Guilford Press.

Ferguson, Iain. 2007. "Neoliberalism, Happiness, and Wellbeing." *International Socialism* 117. http://www.isj.org.uk/index.php4?id=400. Accessed August 5, 2010.

Fisher, Linda. 2000. "Phenomenology and Feminism: Perspectives on Their Relation." In *Feminist Phenomenology*, ed. Linda Fisher and Lester Embree, 17–38. Dordrecht, The Netherlands: Kluwer Academic.

Floyd, Myron F., Kimberly J. Shinew, Francis A. McGuire, and Francis P. Noe. 1994. "Race, Class, and Leisure Activity Preferences: Marginality and Ethnicity Revisited." *Journal of Leisure Research* 26 (2): 158–173.

Flynn, Kristin Joan. 1999. *The Relationship between Body Images and Healthy Eating and Exercise Behaviors among a Sample of Black Women*. Dissertation, Northwestern University.

Foucault, Michel. (1972) 1982. *The Archaeology of Knowledge*. New York: Pantheon.

———. (1977) 1995. *Discipline and Punish: The Birth of the Prison*. New York: Vintage Books.

———. (1981) 1990. *History of Sexuality Volume 1*. New York: Vintage Books.

Frederick, Marla F. 2003. *Between Sundays: Black Women and Everyday Struggles of Faith*. Berkeley: University of California Press.

Freeman, Jo, and Victoria Johnson, ed. 1999. *Waves of Protest: Social Movements since the Sixties*. Boston: Rowman and Littlefield.

Frisby, Cynthia M. 2004. "Does Race Matter? Effects of Idealized Images on African American Women's Perceptions of Body Esteem." *Journal of Black Studies* 34 (3): 323–347.

Gabaccia, Donna R. 1998. *We Are What We Eat: Ethnic Food and the Making of Americans*. Cambridge, Mass.: Harvard University Press.

Galvin, Rose. 2002. "Disturbing Notions of Chronic Illness and Individual Responsibility: Towards a Genealogy of Morals." *Health* 6 (2): 107–137.

Gillespie, Marcia Ann. (1978) 1984. "The Myth of the Strong Black Woman." In *Feminist Frameworks: Alternative Theoretical Accounts of the Relations between Women and Men*, ed. Alison M. Jaggar and Paula S. Rothenberg, 32–35. New York: McGraw-Hill.

Gissendanner, Cindy Himes. 1994. "African American Women in Competitive Sport, 1920–1960." In *Women, Sport, and Culture*, ed. Susan Birrell and Cheryl L. Cole, 81–92. Champaign, Ill.: Human Kinetics.

Gordon, Richard. 1990. *Eating Disorders: Anatomy of a Social Epidemic*. Cambridge, England: Blackwell.

Grady, Denise. 2010. "Obesity Rates Keep Rising, Troubling Health Officials." *New York Times* (August 3). http://www.nytimes.com/2010/08/04/health/ nutrition/04fat.html. Accessed August 4, 2010.

Grant, Jacquelyn. (1979) 1995a. "Black Theology and the Black Woman." In *Words of Fire: An Anthology of African-American Feminist Thought*, ed. Beverly Guy-Sheftall, 320–336. New York: New Press.

———. 1984. "A Black Response to Feminist Theology." In *Women's Spirit Bonding*, ed. Janet Kalven and Mary Buckley, 117–124. New York: Pilgrim Press.

——, ed. 1995b. *Perspectives on Womanist Theology*. Atlanta, Ga.: ITC Press.

Gray, J., K. Ford, and L. Kelly. 1987. "The Prevalence of Bulimia in a Black College Population." *International Journal of Eating Disorders* 6: 753–740.

Gregory, Deborah. 1997. "What's Eating You?" *Essence* 28 (June): 28.

Grossberg, Larry, ed. 1996. "On Postmodernism and Articulation: An Interview with Stuart Hall." Reprinted in *Stuart Hall: Critical Dialogues in Cultural Studies*, ed. David Morley and Kuan-Hsing Chen, 131–150. New York: Routledge.

Grosz, Elizabeth. 1993. "Bodies and Knowledges: Feminism and the Crisis of Reason." In *Feminist Epistemologies*, ed. Linda Alcoff and Elizabeth Potter, 187–216. London: Routledge.

——. 1994. *Volatile Bodies: Toward a Corporeal Feminism*. Bloomington: Indiana University Press.

Guinier, Lani, and Gerald Torres. 2002. *The Miner's Canary: Enlisting Race, Resisting Power, and Transforming Democracy*. Cambridge, Mass.: Harvard University Press.

Hall, Christine C. Iijima. 1995. "Beauty Is in the Soul of the Beholder: Psychological Implications of Beauty and African American Women." *Cultural Diversity and Mental Health* 1 (2): 125–137.

Hall, Stuart. 1985. "Signification, Representation, Ideology: Althusser and the Post-Structuralist Debates." *Critical Studies in Mass Communication* 2 (2): 91–114.

——. (1991) 1997. "Old and New Identities, Old and New Ethnicities." In *Culture, Globalization, and the World-System: Contemporary Conditions for the Representation of Identity*, ed. Anthony D. King, 41–68. Minneapolis: University of Minnesota Press.

——. 1996. "Introduction: Who Needs 'Identity'?" In *Questions of Cultural Identity*, ed. Stuart Hall and Paul du Gay, 1–17. Thousand Oaks, Calif.: Sage.

Haraway, Donna. 1988. "Situated Knowledges: The Science Question in Feminism and the Privilege of Partial Perspective." *Feminist Studies* 14 (3): 575–599.

Harris, Trudier. 1995. "This Disease Called Strength: Some Observations on the Compensating Construction of Black Female Character." *Literature and Medicine* 14: 109–126.

——. 2001. *Saints, Sinners, Saviors: Strong Black Women in African American Literature*. New York: Palgrave.

Harris-Lacewell, Melissa. 2001. "No Place to Rest: African American Political Attitudes and the Myth of Black Women's Strength." *Women and Politics* 23: 1–33.

Hartsock, Nancy. 1985. *Money, Sex, and Power: Toward a Feminist Historical Materialism*. Boston: Northeastern University Press.

———. 1998. *The Feminist Standpoint Revisited and Other Essays*. Boulder, Colo.: Westview Press.

Henderson, Karla A., and Barbara E. Ainsworth. 2001. "Researching Leisure and Physical Activity with Women of Color: Issues and Emerging Questions." *Leisure Sciences* 23 (2): 21–34.

Hewitt, John P. 1998. *The Myth of Self-Esteem: Finding Happiness and Solving Problems in America*. New York: St. Martin's Press.

Heyes, Cressida. (2002) 2007. "Identity Politics." *Stanford Encyclopedia of Philosophy*. http://plato.stanford.edu/entries/identity-politics/. Accessed August 23, 2007.

Heywood, Leslie. 1998. *Bodymakers: A Cultural Anatomy of Women's Bodybuilding*. New Brunswick, N.J.: Rutgers University Press.

Heywood, Leslie, and Shari L. Dworkin. 2003. *Built to Win: The Female Athlete as Cultural Icon*. Minneapolis: University of Minnesota Press.

Holmes, Mary. 2004. "Feeling beyond Rules: Politicizing the Sociology of Emotion and Anger in Feminist Politics." *European Journal of Social Theory* 7 (2): 209–227.

hooks, bell. 1981. *Ain't I a Woman: Black Women and Feminism*. Boston: South End Press.

———. 1990. *Yearning: Race, Gender, and Cultural Politics*. Boston: South End Press.

Jackson, Leslie C., and Beverly Greene, ed. 2000. *Psychotherapy with African American Women: Innovations in Psychodynamic Perspective and Practice*. New York: Guilford Press.

Jones, Jacqueline. (1985) 2010. *Labor of Love, Labor of Sorrow: Black Women, Work, and the Family from Slavery to the Present*, rev. ed. New York: Basic Books.

Jones, James. 1981. *Bad Blood: The Tuskegee Syphilis Experiment*. New York: Free Press.

Kashef, Ziba. 2001. "What We See in the Mirror." *Essence* 31 (April): 96.

King, Deborah. 1993. "Multiple Jeopardy: The Context of a Black Feminist Ideology." In *Feminist Frameworks* (3rd ed.), ed. Alison M. Jaggar and Paula S. Rothenberg, 220–236. New York: McGraw-Hill.

Kingsbury, Kathleen. 2008. "Fit at Any Size." *Time*. http://www.time.com/time/magazine/article/0,9171,1813993,00.htm. Accessed July 28, 2008.

Kruks, Sonia. 2001. *Retrieving Experience: Subjectivity and Recognition in Feminist Politics*. Ithaca, N.Y.: Cornell University Press.

Kumanyika, Shiriki K., and Jeanne B. Charleston. 1992. "Lose Weight and Win: A Church-Based Weight Loss Program for Blood Pressure Control among Black Women." *Patient Education and Counseling* 19: 19–32.

Lacan, Jacques. 1982. "God and the Jouissance of Woman." In *Feminine Sexuality*, ed. Juliet Mitchell and Jacqueline Rose, 137–161. New York: Norton.

———. 2002. *Écrits: A Selection*, trans. Bruce Fink. New York: Norton.

Laclau, Ernesto. 1977. *Politics and Ideology in Marxist Theory*. London: New Left Books.

Laclau, Ernesto, and Chantal Mouffe. 1985. *Hegemony and Socialist Strategy: Towards a Radical Democratic Politics*, trans. W. Moore and P. Cammack. London: Verso.

Lansbury, Jennifer H. 2001. "'The Tuskegee Flash' and 'the Slender Harlem Stroker': Black Women Athletes on the Margin." *Journal of Sport History* 28 (2): 233–252.

Larana, Enrique, Hank Johnston, and Joseph R. Gusfield, ed. 1994. *New Social Movements: From Ideology to Identity*. Philadelphia: Temple University Press.

Littlejohn, Eugia Monique. 1994. *The Relationship between the Components of Black Feminism and Psychological Health in African American Women*. Dissertation, Ohio State University.

Logio, Kim A. 2003. "Gender, Race, Childhood Abuse, and Body Image among Adolescents." *Violence against Women* 9 (8): 931–954.

Lorde, Audre. 1984. *Sister Outsider: Essays and Speeches*. Berkeley, Calif.: Crossing Press.

Lovejoy, Meg. 2001. "Disturbances in the Social Body: Differences in Body Image and Eating Problems among African American and White Women." *Gender and Society* 15 (2): 239–261.

Lubiano, Wahneema. 1992. "Black Ladies, Welfare Queens, and State Minstrels: Ideological War by Narrative Means." In *Race-ing Justice, En-Gendering Power: Essays on Anita Hill, Clarence Thomas, and the Construction of Social Reality*, ed. Toni Morrison, 323–363. New York: Pantheon.

Lupton, Deborah. 1995. *The Imperative of Health: Public Health and the Regulated Body*. London: Sage.

Majeed, Debra Mubashshir. 2006. "Response" to Monica A. Coleman's "Must I Be a Womanist?" *Journal of Feminist Studies in Religion* 22 (1): 113–118.

Marshall, Helen. 1996. "Our Bodies Ourselves: Why We Should Add Old Fashioned Empirical Phenomenology to the New Theories of the Body." *Women's Studies International Forum* 19 (3): 253–265.

Martin, Jane Roland. 1994. "Methodological Essentialism, False Difference, and Other Dangerous Traps." *Signs* 19 (3): 630–657.

Martin, Joan. 1978. "Church Women and the Women's Movement: Speaking Out from a Black Perspective." *Church Woman* (November): 11–13.

Matsuda, Mari J. 1996. *Where Is Your Body? And Other Essays on Race, Gender, and the Law*. Boston: Beacon Press.

Matsuda, Mari J., Charles R. Lawrence III, Richard Delgado, and Kimberlé Crenshaw, ed. 1993. *Words That Wound: Critical Race Theory, Assaultive Speech, and the First Amendment*. Boulder, Colo.: Westview Press.

Mattis, Jacqueline S. 1995. *Work(I)ngs of the Spirit: Spirituality, Meaning Construction, and Coping in the Lives of Black Women.* Dissertation, University of Michigan.

McGregor, Sue. 2001. "Neoliberalism and Health Care." *International Journal of Consumer Studies* 25 (2): 82–89.

McKay, Nellie Y. 1989. "Nineteenth Century Black Women's Spiritual Autobiographies: Religious Faith and Self-Empowerment." In *Interpreting Women's Lives*, ed. Joy Webster Barbre, 139–154. Bloomington: Indiana University Press.

Mintz, Sidney W., and Christine M. Du Bois. 2002. "The Anthropology of Food and Eating." *Annual Review of Anthropology* 31: 99–119.

Mitchell, Angela, and Kennise Herring. 1998. *What the Blues Is All About.* New York: Perigee Trade.

Mitchem, Stephanie Y. 2006. "Response" to Monica A. Coleman's "Must I Be a Womanist?" *Journal of Feminist Studies in Religion* 22 (1): 123–128.

Moglen, Helene. 2008. "Ageing and Transageing: Transgenerational Hauntings of the Self." *Studies in Gender and Sexuality* 9 (4): 297–311.

Mohanty, Satya P. 1993. "The Epistemic Status of Cultural Identity: On 'Beloved' and the Postcolonial Condition." *Cultural Critique* 24 (Spring): 41–80.

Monroe, Irene. 2006. "Response" to Monica A. Coleman's "Must I Be a Womanist?" *Journal of Feminist Studies in Religion* 22 (1): 107–113.

Moraga, Cherríe. 1983. *Loving in the War Years: Lo que nunca pasó por sus labios.* Boston: South End Press.

Murray, Pauli. 1979. "Black Theology and Feminist Theology." In *Black Theology: A Documentary History*, ed. Gayraud S. Wilmore and James H. Cone, 304–322. Maryknoll, N.Y.: Orbis Books.

Nelson, Diane. 1999. *A Finger in the Wound: Body Politics in Quincentennial Guatemala.* Berkeley: University of California Press.

Neustadt, Kathy. 1992. *Clambake: A History and Celebration of an American Tradition.* Boston: University of Massachusetts Press.

Offe, Claus. 1985. "New Social Movements: Challenging the Boundaries of Institutional Politics." *Social Research* 52 (4): 817–868.

Oliver, J. Eric. 2006. *Fat Politics: The Real Story behind America's Obesity Epidemic.* Oxford, England: Oxford University Press.

Penkal, Jessica Lynn, and Lawrence A. Kurdek. 2007. "Gender and Race Differences in Young Adults' Body Dissatisfaction." *Personality and Individual Differences* 43 (8): 2270–2281.

Phillips, Crystal J., and Deborah Gregory. 1997. "Weighting to Exhale." *Essence* 28 (June): 26–30.

Pilcher, Jeffrey M. 1998. *Que Vivan los Tamales! Food and the Making of Mexican Identity.* Albuquerque: University of New Mexico Press.

Powell, Lisa M., Sandy Slater, Frank J. Chaloupka, and Deborah Harper. 2006. "Availability of Physical Activity–Related Facilities and Neighborhood Demographic and Socioeconomic Characteristics: A National Study." *American Journal of Public Health* 96 (9): 1676–1680.

Powers, Retha. 1989. "Fat Is a Black Women's Issue." *Essence* 20 (October): 75–78, 134–136.

Rand, Colleen S., and John M. Kuldah. 1990. "The Epidemiology of Obesity and Self-Defined Weight Problems in the General Population: Gender, Race, and Social Class." *International Journal of Eating Disorders* 9: 329–343.

Rapping, Elayne. 1996. *The Culture of Recovery: Making Sense of the Self-Help Movement in Women's Lives.* New York: Beacon Press.

Razak, Arisika. 2006. "Response" to Monica A. Coleman's "Must I Be a Womanist?" *Journal of Feminist Studies in Religion* 22 (1): 100–107.

Reverby, Susan. 2009. *Examining Tuskegee: The Infamous Syphilis Study and Its Legacy.* Chapel Hill: University of North Carolina Press.

Riggs, Marcia Y. 1994. *Awake, Arise, and Act: A Womanist Call for Black Liberation.* Cleveland, Ohio: Pilgrim Press.

Roberts, Alan, Thomas F. Cash, Alan Feingold, and Blair T. Johnson. 2006. "Are Black-White Differences in Females' Body Dissatisfaction Decreasing? A Meta-Analytic Review." *Journal of Counseling and Clinical Psychology* 74 (6): 1121–1131.

Romero, Regina E. 2000. "The Icon of the Strong Black Woman: The Paradox of Strength." In *Psychotheraphy with African American Women: Innovations in Psychodynamic Perspective and Practice,* ed. Leslie C. Jackson and Beverly Greene, 225–238. New York: Guilford Press.

Rose, Tricia. 2003. *Longing to Tell: Black Women Talk about Sexuality and Intimacy.* New York: Picador.

Salih, Sara, with Judith Butler, ed. 2004. *The Judith Butler Reader.* Malden, Mass.: Blackwell.

Sandoval, Chela. 2000. *Methodology of the Oppressed.* Minneapolis: University of Minnesota Press.

Scheman, Naomi. 1980. "Anger and the Politics of Naming." In *Women and Language in Literature and Society,* ed. Sally McConnell-Ginet, Ruth Borker, and Nelly Furman, 174–187. New York: Praeger.

Scott, Joan W. 1991. "The Evidence of Experience." *Critical Inquiry* 17 (4): 773–797.

Scruggs, Afi-Odelia. 2001. "Media and Our Mind-Set." *Essence* 31 (April): 94.

Shaw, Heather, Lisa Ramirez, Ariel Trost, Pat Randall, and Eric Stice. 2004. "Body Image and Eating Disturbances across Ethnic Groups: More Similarities Than Differences." *Psychology of Addictive Behaviors* 18: 12–8.

Shelton, Deborah L. 2001. "A Perfectly Healthy Body." *Essence* 31 (April): 98.

Shinew, Kimberly J., Myron F. Floyd, Francis A. McGuire, and Francis P. Noe. 1995. "Gender, Race, and Subjective Social Class and Their Association with Leisure Preferences." *Leisure Sciences* 17 (2): 75–89.

Shortridge, Barbara G., and James R. Shortridge, ed. 1998. *The Taste of American Place: A Reader on Regional and Ethnic Foods.* Lanham, Md.: Rowman and Littlefield.

Siegel, Judith M., Antronette K. Yancey, and William J. McCarthy. 2000. "Overweight and Depressive Symptoms among African-American Women." *Preventive Medicine* 31: 232–240.

Sklar, Deidre. 1994. "Can Bodylore Be Brought to Its Senses?" *Journal of American Folklore* 107 (423): 9–22.

Skye, Lee Miena. 2006. "Response" to Monica A. Coleman's "Must I Be a Womanist?" *Journal of Feminist Studies in Religion* 22 (1): 119–123.

Slack, Jennifer Daryl. 1996. "The Theory and Method of Articulation." In *Stuart Hall: Critical Dialogues in Cultural Studies*, ed. David Morley and Kuan-Hsing Chen, 112–127. New York: Routledge.

Smith, Susan L. 1995. *Sick and Tired of Being Sick and Tired: Black Women's Health Activism in America, 1890–1950.* Philadelphia: University of Pennsylvania Press.

Smith, Valerie. 1998. *Not Just Race, Not Just Gender: Black Feminist Readings.* New York: Routledge.

Smith, Yevonne. 1992. "Women of Color in Society and Sport." *Quest* 44 (2): 228–250.

Spelman, Elizabeth V. 1989. "Anger and Insubordination." In *Women, Knowledge, and Reality*, ed. Ann Garry and Marilyn Pearsall, 263–274. New York: Routledge.

Spivak, Gayatri. 1987. *In Other Worlds: Essays in Cultural Politics.* New York: Taylor and Francis.

Steinem, Gloria. 1992. *The Revolution from Within: A Book of Self-Esteem.* New York: Little, Brown.

Stephenson, Frank. 2004. "For the Love of 'ME.'" *Florida State University Research in Review* (Summer): 16–31.

Studlar, Gaylyn. 1990. "Reconciling Feminism and Phenomenology: Notes on Problems and Possibilities, Texts and Contexts." *Quarterly Review of Film and Video* 12 (3): 69–78.

Tarrow, Sidney. 1994. *Power in Movement: Collective Action, Social Movements and Politics.* Cambridge, England: Cambridge University Press.

Thomas, Anita Jones, Karen McCurtis Witherspoon, and Suzette L. Speight. 2004. "Toward the Development of the Stereotypic Roles for Black Women Scale." *Journal of Black Psychology* 30 (3): 426–441.

Thompson, Becky W. 1994. *A Hunger So Wide and So Deep: American Women Speak Out on Eating Problems.* Minneapolis: University of Minnesota Press.

Thompson, Cheryl L. 2000. "African American Women and Moral Masochism: When There Is Too Much of a Good Thing." In *Psychotherapy with African American Women: Innovations in Psychodynamic Perspectives and Practice*, ed. Leslie C. Jackson and Beverly Greene, 239–250. New York: Guilford Press.

Thompson, Sharon H., and Roger G. Sargent. 2000. "Black and White Women's Weight-Related Attitudes and Parental Criticism of Their Childhood Appearance." *Women and Health* 30 (3): 77–92.

Tilly, Charles. 1978. *From Mobilization to Revolution*. Reading, Mass.: Addison-Wesley.

———. 2004. *Social Movements, 1768–2004*. Boulder, Colo.: Paradigm.

Townes, Emilie M. 1995. *In a Blaze of Glory: Womanist Spirituality as Social Witness*. Nashville, Tenn.: Abingdon Press.

———. 1998. *Breaking the Fine Rain of Death: African American Health Issues and a Womanist Ethic of Care*. New York: Continuum.

U.S. Department of Health and Human Services, Agency for Healthcare Research and Quality. 2009. "National Healthcare Disparities Report." AHRQ Publication No. 10-0004 (March 2010).

Vertinsky, Patricia, and Gwendolyn Captain. 1998. "More Myth Than History: American Culture and Representations of the Black Female's Athletic Ability." *Journal of Sport History* 25 (3): 532–561.

Walker, Alice. 1983. *In Search of Our Mothers' Gardens: Womanist Prose*. New York: Harcourt Brace Jovanovich.

Wallace, Michelle. (1990) 1978. *Black Macho and the Myth of the Superwoman*. New York: Verso.

Ward, Steven. 1996. "Filling the World with Self-Esteem: A Social History of Truth-Making." *Canadian Journal of Sociology* 21 (1): 1–23.

Warren, Barbara Jones. 1997. "Depression, Stressful Life Events, Social Support, and Self-Esteem in Middle Class African American Women." *Archives of Psychiatric Nursing* 11 (3): 107–117.

Weathers, Diane. 2003a. "Our Bodies, Ourselves." *Essence* 34 (September): 28.

———. 2003b. "Why Diets Alone Don't Work." *Essence* 34 (September): 188–194.

Wells, C. L. 1996. "Physical Activity and Women's Health." *Physical Activity and Fitness Research Digest* (March): 1–8.

West, Traci C. 1999. *Wounds of the Spirit: Black Women, Violence, and Resistance Ethics*. New York: New York University Press.

———. 2006. "Response" to Monica A. Coleman's "Must I Be a Womanist?" *Journal of Feminist Studies in Religion* 22 (1): 128–134.

Williams, Patricia J. 1991. *The Alchemy of Race and Rights: A Diary of a Law Professor*. Cambridge, Mass.: Harvard University Press.

Williams-Forson, Psyche A. 2006. *Building Houses out of Chicken Legs: Black Women, Food, and Power*. Chapel Hill: University of North Carolina Press.

Woods-Giscombé, Cheryl L. 2010. "Superwoman Schema: African American Women's Views on Stress, Strength, and Health." *Qualitative Health Research* 20 (5): 668–683.

Young, D. R., K. W. Miller, L. B. Wilder, L. R. Yanek, and D. M. Becker. 1998. "Physical Activity Patterns of Urban African Americans." *Journal of Community Health* 23 (2): 99–112.

Young, Iris. 1980. "Throwing Like a Girl: A Phenomenology of Feminine Body Comportment, Motility, and Spatiality." *Human Studies* 3 (1): 137–156.

Index

Kimberly J. Lau is Professor of Literature and American Studies at the University of California, Santa Cruz. She is the author of *New Age Capitalism: Making Money East of Eden*.

.

Printed by Printforce, United Kingdom